ROUTLEDGE LIBRARY EDITIONS:
BRITISH SOCIOLOGICAL
ASSOCIATION

Volume 16

LOCATING HEALTH

LOCATING HEALTH

Sociological and historical explorations

Edited by
STEPHEN PLATT, HILARY THOMAS,
SUE SCOTT AND GARETH WILLIAMS

Routledge
Taylor & Francis Group
LONDON AND NEW YORK

First published in 1993 by Avebury Ashgate Publishing Limited

This edition first published in 2018
by Routledge
2 Park Square, Milton Park, Abingdon, Oxon OX14 4RN

and by Routledge
711 Third Avenue, New York, NY 10017

Routledge is an imprint of the Taylor & Francis Group, an informa business

British Library Cataloguing in Publication Data
A catalogue record for this book is available from the British Library

ISBN: 978-1-138-49942-3 (Set)
ISBN: 978-1-351-01463-2 (Set) (ebk)
ISBN: 978-0-8153-4862-7 (Volume 16) (hbk)
ISBN: 978-1-351-16640-9 (Volume 16) (ebk)

Locating Health

Sociological and historical explorations

Edited by

STEPHEN PLATT
HILARY THOMAS
SUE SCOTT
GARETH WILLIAMS

Explorations in Sociology No. 44

Avebury
Aldershot • Brookfield USA • Hong Kong • Singapore • Sydney

Published by
Avebury
Ashgate Publishing Limited
Gower House
Croft Road
Aldershot
Hants GU11 3HR
England

Ashgate Publishing Company
Old Post Road
Brookfield
Vermont 05036
USA

British Library Cataloguing in Publication Data

Locating Health: Sociological and Historical
Explorations – (Explorations in Sociology Series;
No. 44)
I. Platt, Stephen II. Series
306.4

ISBN 1 85628 367 4

Details of other volumes in the *Explorations in Sociology* series are available from:

British Sociological Association Publications
Unit 3G, Mountjoy Research Centre
Stockton Road
Durham DH1 3SW

Printed and Bound in Great Britain by
Athenaeum Press Ltd, Newcastle upon Tyne.

Contents

List of figures

List of tables

Acknowledgements

Many people have supported the production of this volume, but our main thanks go to two people: Anne Dix, the British Sociological Association's Administrative Secretary whose knowledge, organizational skill and support made organizing the BSA's 1991 conference a much more pleasant experience than it would otherwise have been; and Nick Dalziel, the BSA's Publications Officer, for the hard work he has put into negotiating the publication of this volume.

Foreword

Uta Gerhardt
University of Giessen, Germany

Over the last decade, health has become a major focus of medical sociological thinking. This book shows the high quality of studies addressing this issue. In most contributions, as in most research so far, the loss or failure of health, that is, illness or premature death, is analysed in terms of the differences between the genders, social classes, regions or Eastern and Western countries. Indirectly, a theoretical question is approached (What is the societal nature of health?) and tackled through investigation of ill health using research which maps out where health is absent, and why, and in which societies.

My remarks in this foreword supplement the standpoint outlined for sociology by the various contributions to this book. To that question, What is the sociological nature of health? I can only sketch a tentative answer. It stands at the beginning of this book, providing a conceptual baseline for the argument substantiated by the chapters below. The reader may keep it in mind while reading the chapters, and judge at the end whether or not it provides a useful framework for reconciling the medical sociological endeavour with general sociology.

Behind sociology's attempts to embrace health as the epitome of equality of life-chances in society, may be seen seminal changes of modern democracy's moral constitution. The French Revolution, based on the ideas of secular morality in enlightenment philosophy, built democracy on the principles of political freedom, equality and fraternity. The virtues and communalities of the *citizen* became the apex of a democratic world. Liberty, equality and fraternity were to be realized through political process and institutions guaranteeing division of power and human rights. Absolutism was to be overcome through constitutional and judicial controls that protected the individual against encroachments of the state upon life and liberty.

In the course of the nineteenth and first half of the twentieth centuries in Europe, the emergence of socialism changed the scene. It made clear that the French Revolution's accomplishment of republicanism did not go far enough to satisfy the tenet of social justice inherent in the philosophy of democracy. While liberty, equality and fraternity were proclaimed as ideals, most of the population continued to suffer from want, and to be submitted to merciless exploitation of their powerlessness. Thus, it was on the level of the individual as *bourgeois* that democracy became imperative. Socialism proclaimed freedom, equality and fraternity (community) among individuals as productive participants of the economy. By striving to overcome the class structure that institutionalizes the dichotomy between the haves and the have-nots of means of production, society was to turn into a fully-fledged democracy in more than the political sense.

In the second half of the twentieth century, however, new aspects of the ubiquitous lack of freedom and hitherto unnoticed bias in fraternity have been recognized. At the same time, inequality is found to remain unconquered. After an era of two world wars and of historically unrivalled denial of human beings' right to life under German national socialism, a third dimension of democracy has gradually emerged as a viable tenet.

The scene was set, in the 1960s, by anti-psychiatry's revelations about the banalities of power behind the absurdities of so-called custodial care as treatment for mental illness. A relevant *weltanschauung* emerged, namely Foucault's philosophy of mentality. He focused on 'docile bodies' submitted to administrative surveillance that domesticates their lust and habituates their lesions (Foucault 1963, 1975). The body came to attract philosophy's and sociology's interest, particularly inasmuch as it epitomized society's lack of freedom, failure to establish equality, and unquestioned discrimination or unabated competitive individualism, instead of fraternity. It was the greatest injustice imaginable that not only conditions of life, but life-spans themselves should differ by social membership, that is, be cut short for the disenfranchised. The alternative was health for all, provided by the guarantor of equality for all classes, if only on principle, namely, the welfare state.

In this connection some sociologists have come to criticize, with the aim of responsibly counteracting, the medicalization of society. The idea is that the dominant model of deviance has changed 'from badness to sickness', to use Schneider and Conrad's phrase, and treatment has replaced punishment as the mode of correction (Conrad and Schneider 1980). This accords autonomy and power to the medical profession to an unprecedented degree. Doctors are depicted as constructing – if not inventing – the catalogue of nosological categories governing diagnosis and treatment. Yet their supremacy appears to hinder rather than facilitate health for all. Their power of definition concerning diagnosis of illness is said to increase, albeit inadvertently, inequality and discrimination in respect of life chances or quality of life. Progress is envisaged, on the one hand, through a broadening of the scope of medical knowledge to include less technical and non-hospital based care. On the other hand, social support and other forms of self-help are invited into the realm of medical practice benefiting the patient as a person.

In denouncing uncontrolled medical dominance over health care, however, sociology unwittingly finds itself compelled to underwrite the position and politics of the state. This becomes more difficult now after the collapse of Eastern European communist welfare states, exposing in their wake practices of false statistics, inhuman hospital routines, impersonal care as well as political pressure on doctors deprived of professional autonomy but submitted to surveillance by secret police and party officials. This reveals that state domination over structure and delivery of health care can be as power-oriented as professional domination, despite the fact that the representatives of power are bureaucrats rather than doctors, and their logic is administrative, fiscal and that of party politics, rather than clinical.

In the irrefutable interest of democracy and equality for the sake of the patient, sociology often turns against the medical profession. In contrast, Durkheim and Parsons considered the professions suitable guarantors of democracy and equality, inasmuch as relationships between physician and patient should require the former's utmost competence and universalist principles (Durkheim [1895] 1933; Parsons 1975). By turning to the state and rejecting professional responsibility for health equity, sociology might inadvertently back the forces apt to destroy professional independence, possibly one of the last bastions of non-state surveilled institutional care and (self) control in society.

This leaves medical sociology with the problem of having discovered a realm where progress is definitely called for, but backing forces of apparent progress that may lead in the direction of societal regression. Parsons analysed German national socialism and also soviet communism as regressive societies that had lapsed back from a rational–legal to a traditional (patrimonial) type of authority (Gerhardt 1993). Independent professions setting their own responsible norms of practice indebted to human need and suffering, and free from economic considerations, epitomized for Parsons a society most apt to fulfil the human condition (Parsons 1978). Sociology has rightly pointed out that prevailing inequalities in health and life prospects represent an element of traditionalism not hitherto analysed in general social theory. But the question is whether overcoming professional dominance and establishing an all-pervasive welfare state is an adequate means to this end, or whether it serves to strengthen rather than supercede elements in present-day society.

This dilemma is so intricate, in my view, that research in medical sociology is right not to face it head-on. Rather, newly available data from Eastern Europe reveal all-pervasive repression and inequality in the allegedly well-organized and equitable communist welfare state(s). This is now documented together with similar traditionalism in the West. Thus, ill-health is shown to pervade society in certain sectors whose deprivation has long been ideologically camouflaged for false pride of progress. Virchow's observation in 1848 that typhoid fever and poverty form a vicious circle, has lost little of its acumen (Virchow 1849).

However, health, as the World Health Organization has maintained for over forty years, is more than the absence of illness. According to the well-known definition spurred by post-World War II enthusiasm for enduring peace and universal well-being, it includes psychological as well as social conditions of life. From this perspective, health is partly utopian as a state of the person or body suggesting optimal inner and outer mastery.

As such an all-encompassing scope of being, health is near impossible to delineate in research. Even if levels of health are distinguished, and even if objective or clinical health is separated from subjective or experienced health, the problem remains methodologically treacherous. It is unclear what measurement could integrate social, psychological, and physiological functioning or well-being in a way meaningful to the researcher who refuses to settle for nominal definitions that he or she simply applies to the empirical world. Above all, research focusing on health must be able to interpret its results or outcomes in a way that allows insights into social reality and may even benefit social theory or some parts of society at large.

In this vein, Parsons warns that the WHO's definition of health is misguided. Although health incorporates an organic as well as an action level, and therefore physical and social aspects, he claims it is related to the 'problem of meaning of this life and its vicissitudes' (Parsons 1978:81) in a way different from politics. The societal ideal of universally decent living conditions applies differently to health and to political participation. According to Parsons, well-being in general encompasses an individual's control over his or her inner as well as outer environment. Failure of well-being in case of illness, however, is not due to a person's lack of willpower to control his self or his environment. He therefore opts for a less inclusive conception of health in order to enable social science to tackle successfully the relevant problem areas by research and analysis. 'Of course,' he writes, 'in the spheres of ego function, of voluntary action, the degree of control open to any particular individual is always limited by conditions beyond his control, such as those altogether outside human (certainly individual) control (e.g. the weather) and those in the control of other human agencies (as in the much discussed sphere of power relations). This sphere of uncontrolled factors includes exposure to risk of the genesis of illness. To identify "powerlessness" in this sense with illness is, however, highly confusing. They are quite different aspects of the human predicament' (Parsons 1978:81).

'Locating health', from this vantage point, is an empirical as well as a theoretical endeavour. Discussion of the societal nature of health has been conducted among medical sociologists for some two decades, and seriously during only the last few years. It may well become the central topic in medical sociology towards the year 2000.

References

Conrad, Peter and Schneider, Joseph W. (1980), *Deviance and Medicalization: From badness to sickness*, St. Louis: Mosby.

Durkheim, Emile (1933), *On the Division of Labour in Society*, New York: Macmillan (originally 1895).

Foucault, Michel (1973), *The Birth of the Clinic: An archaeology of medical perception*, London: Tavistock (originally 1963).

Foucault, Michel (1978), *Discipline and Punish. The Birth of the Prison*, New York: Random House (originally 1975).

Gerhardt, Uta (1989), *Ideas About Illness: An intellectual and political history of medical sociology*, London: Macmillan.

Gerhardt, Uta (ed.), (1993), *Talcott Parsons On National Socialism*, New York: Aldine.

Parsons, Talcott (1975), 'The sick role and role of the physician reconsidered', *Milbank Memorial Fund Health and Society*, **53**:257–278.

Parsons, Talcott (1978), 'Health and disease: a sociological and action perspective', in: *Action Theory and the Human Condition*, London: Free Press, pp. 68–81.

Virchow, Rudolf (1849), 'Mitteilungen über die in Oberschlesien herrschende Typhus-Epidemie: Archiv für pathologische Anatomie und Physiologie und für klinische Medizin', **2**:143–322. (Report on the current typhoid epidemic in Upper Silesia. Reprinted from the original, Hildesheim: Georg Ohms Verlagsbuchhandlung 1968.)

1 Introduction

Stephen Platt and Hilary Thomas

Health divisions and inequalities have been long-standing topics of empirical investigation and interpretation among sociologists, epidemiologists and those charged with promoting and maintaining the public health. During the last decade alone several books and edited collections, as well as countless articles in academic journals, have been devoted to describing, measuring and explaining variations in morbidity and mortality by class and economic activity. Nevertheless, a number of lacunae or weak spots in the health inequalities debate can still be identified. These include the relative neglect of divisions associated with other key social locations, such as gender, age and race/ethnicity, and the overemphasis on mortality, which is increasingly recognized as a poor indicator of morbidity and an even less adequate guide to positive health. Furthermore, there has been a failure to devise and execute sound empirical tests of competing explanations for the (widening) health inequalities which are uncovered; and an increasing disjunction between advances in statistical techniques and methodological sophistication, on the one hand, and underdeveloped conceptual and theoretical frameworks, on the other.

The chapters in this collection are revised versions of papers originally presented at the British Sociological Association's 1991 conference, entitled 'Health and Society'. The balance of the collection attempts to shift the existing debate towards a consideration of some of the complexities of health inequalities research by addressing issues of morbidity rather than mortality, emphasizing the theoretical and conceptual bases of the subject and developing new methodological approaches in the examination of data. Four major concerns can be identified throughout the collection: the reconceptualization of key theoretical terms; the health consequences of multiple social locations; the reciprocal relationships between different locations; and the importance of newly identified social locations. Much of the discussion about inequalities in health has taken occupational social class as a framework for the social differentiation of circumstances and resources within the population. Within this collection the importance of income differentials is subjected to detailed scrutiny. Likewise, the boundaries of paid employment are assessed in relation to both domestic labour and retirement. The direct implications of paid employment for the health of workers are considered. The need to clarify similar constructs within different social structures is highlighted by an analysis of gender and health in Eastern and Western Europe. Early retirement provides a salient focus for an examination of the reciprocal influence of health and social location. The complexity of understanding multiple location within social structure is addressed in chapters combining gender and class, and gender and age. Newly emergent locations include place, consumption and 'lifestyle'.

Richard Wilkinson draws attention to the highly significant correlation between income distribution and average life expectancy in the developed countries and, having dismissed the likelihood of reverse causation or spurious association, concludes that 'relative income does indeed affect health'. On the basis of further empirical analysis he concludes that it is the social meanings of structural inequality ('how we stand in relation to each other'), rather than the physical effects of poverty ('where we stand in terms of any absolute standards'), which may now have a significant impact upon our physical and emotional well-being. Although the pathway between income distribution and death is as yet little understood, Wilkinson suggests that we need to explore further the role of psychosocial risk factors, in particular reduced or inadequate social affiliations (poor social support, lack of confiding relationship), which in turn may be linked to behavioural risk factors, such as smoking or alcohol/drug abuse.

Sara Arber and Jay Ginn analyse the ways in which three types of resources – the health and physical abilities of the individual and other household members; material or structural resources, such as income and housing; and access to personal, supportive and health care – interlock to form a 'resource triangle' which influences independence, well-being and personal space among people aged 65 years and over. Their chapter examines the inter-relationships between these three sets of resources and demonstrates how the resource triangle is gendered, with older women being systematically disadvantaged in each of the three key resources compared to older men. However, the authors also note that gender differences in self-assessed health in later life appear to be less important than differences associated with class. They comment that the finding of strong class gradients:

> may be surprising, given that for elderly people occupational class is based on their labour market position many years earlier, especially for women of this generation who may not have worked since marriage.

Overall they conclude that the resource triangle is affected by both gender and class: elderly women and working-class elderly people suffer the most unfavourable conditions in each kind of resource. The inequalities caused during the economically active years by disadvantageous locations in the productive and reproductive systems form part of the burden that is carried into old age.

Sally Macintyre compares Western European (and North American) data on gender differences in longevity and health with new data now emerging from Eastern European countries. Life expectancy at one year of age is about four years higher in the West, and the difference in longevity between men and women is greater in the East. Between the mid-1960s and the mid-1980s, when life expectancy was increasing in Western Europe, there was actually a decline in life expectancy in a number of east European countries (USSR, Romania, Bulgaria, Hungary, Czechoslovakia and Poland). Macintyre laments the artificial separation between the literature on health inequalities and the literature on gender differences in health. The latter reveals the well-known paradox that, while women are more likely to suffer from illness and disability, and to use more health care resources, men die at a younger age. Noting that the body of knowledge concerning gender differences in illness and disability mainly originates in empirical studies conducted in North America and Western Europe, Macintyre speculates whether the current explanations based on the expectation of gender-segregated roles are likely to be as applicable to the situation in Eastern Europe. She concludes with a plea for the incorporation of gender differentials in morbidity and mortality into research and thinking about social inequalities in health.

An historical perspective to debates about women's employment and the relationship to domestic labour is provided by Barbara Harrison. She seeks to explore the health consequences of women's working conditions in late nineteenth-century and early twentieth-century Britain, in particular the significance of occupational health as a issue within feminist analysis and politics. By the 1840s state intervention in the industrial system (by means of 'protective' legislation) included women as well as children in its purview. Harrison demonstrates that the protection of women as a special group arose out of concerns about their continuing ability to care for their husbands and children (domestic role) as well as worries about their perceived physical vulnerability. The intention of factory legislation, however, was not necessarily to protect the health of women *qua* workers, but to protect the health of the nation from the dangers of working women by preserving separate gendered domains of responsibility and women's duty to preserve the health of others within their domestic role.

Jennie Popay and Mel Bartley develop an integrated theory of the relationships between labour conditions, gender and social class inequalities in health. Using a proportional odds modelling technique and data from two national datasets, they explore the relative importance of domestic working conditions in shaping the experience of ill-health among women in paid employment. After controlling for the effect of long-term health status, new measures of domestic conditions and physical and psychosocial conditions of formal paid work (employment) were associated with a significant increase in the risk of experiencing severe recent illness among women. Among men, however, no such effects were found. More importantly, perhaps, conventional measures of working conditions – namely, class and employment status – failed to make a significant independent contribution to the models. Although the authors rightly voice their concern about the validity of the short-term health measures used in the analysis, we endorse their claims for the theoretical significance of unified measures of labour demands and conditions.

Whereas early retirement used to be connected almost exclusively to deteriorating health, recent commentators have suggested that economic/financial factors may now be more salient. Based on a review of the evidence from three recent studies of male early retirement, Dallas Cliff argues that, while the majority of early retirees have responded to favourably perceived economic incentives, a substantial minority of men, mainly manual workers, are replicating earlier patterns by taking early retirement due to a breakdown in health:

> [W]hile most early retirees go on to negotiate varied careers which mix family and leisure pursuits, short-term and part-time employment and voluntary work in ways that are generally highly satisfying, others, mainly manual workers, experience early retirement in terms of ill-health careers that cut down their options and leave them financially and socially impoverished.

Cliff finds empirical support for the contention that the divide between 'lifestyle-orientated' (mainly middle class) retirees and those who are reproducing earlier patterns of health-related early retirement (mainly working class) is widening.

In an historical case study Andrew Watterson looks at the introduction of new technologies into the gas industry in the late nineteenth and early twentieth centuries, the occupational health hazards created by such developments, and the responses of workers and other key groups. He concludes that, although gas workers tried to combat the prevailing ignorance about occupational ill-health in the industry, they were:

> neither able to alter the dominant established social processes for defining occupational diseases nor overcome the political economy of the time which created particular gas industry health hazards.... Occupational medicine lost the struggle to political economy at an early date.

In his chapter Peter Phillimore seeks to wean the debate about inequalities in health away from its excessive reliance on simple statistical measures and the epidemiological paradigm, towards a broader sociological understanding of the social creation of health differences. He starts with evidence of excessive mortality in the poorer and predominantly working-class areas of Middlesbrough compared to that found in similarly constituted areas of neighbouring Sunderland. Based on the proposition that, whatever the broad socio-economic similarities between the two populations, 'there must also be striking differences in the lives people lead in these towns to have produced such dissimilar mortality patterns', Phillimore sets out to examine three sociological themes that may be relevant to an understanding of such differences: the industrial environment, polarization and social inequality within each town, and 'the ways in which people themselves shape their environment in the two towns'. When, in the context of this third theme, Phillimore refers to 'lifestyle', he does not have in mind disparate individualized behaviours such as smoking or drinking, but rather 'fears, values and habits', the conceptualization of 'daily routines, decision-making and choice against a background of a struggle to survive'.

In his contribution to the debate about the costs and benefits of the industrial revolution to the well-being of the British population, Rory Williams examines the regional health experience of historical and contemporary Clydeside and presents an initial assessment of the role of immigration from the Scottish Highlands and from Ireland in Clydeside's industrialization. Whereas in England falling prices after the Napoleonic War tended to lead to a rise in real wages, the reverse was true in Clydeside. Moreover, although Glasgow's death rate was only slightly higher than the English national figure in 1821, the ensuing rise in industrial output and surge of immigration was accompanied by a rapidly escalating death rate which did not fall back to the 1821 level until over 60 years later; over the same period the death rate in England remained fairly steady. Williams argues that the growth of industrialism coincided with the collapse of peasant populations, and that the mortality profile of Glasgow and Clydeside was related to 'patterns of urban poverty brought about by the migration and factors antecedent and subsequent to it'.

Michael Calnan, Sarah Cant and Jonathan Gabe draw on recently collected data on private health insurance in order to examine the theories of consumption in relation to health care. In particular, they ask whether the development of private health insurance signifies 'new' social divisions (in distinction to traditional divisions, such as social class, relating to the sphere of production). On the basis of qualitative interviews with 60 middle-aged men (of whom 20 had chosen to take out private health insurance, 20 had been co-opted into employer-run schemes, and 20 who had not subscribed to a scheme), the authors conclude that:

> consumption of private health insurance has little power to explain or account for the 'new' social divisions.... [T]he evidence from this study adds weight to the claims of those who have argued that private medical care challenges the proposition that divisions of consumption have replaced divisions of production.

In the final chapter David Smith and Malcolm Nicolson consider twentieth-century discourse about the diet of the working class and show that recent allegations of ignorance constitute merely another example of a moralizing rhetoric used repeatedly by scientists and politicians. They argue that the association of ignorance with ill-health is:

> both a structured ideological response to the social threats and dangers posed by class inequality and a feature of the general pattern of control and discipline imposed upon the body in an advanced industrial society.

The chapters in *Locating Health* are intended to make a stimulating intellectual contribution to the debate on health-related divisions and inequalities which is likely to continue unabated during the 1990s. While the issues covered in this book are undoubtedly of interest to academics teaching or researching in the sociology of health and illness, it is hoped that policy planners will find the collection of practical relevance in the implementation of recent health care reforms, especially the identification of health needs within special population subgroups.

2 The impact of income inequality on life expectancy

Richard G. Wilkinson

Introduction

When I first got involved in research on 'inequalities' – or social class differences – in health, I was sensitive to the charge that the issue was really only of interest to those who were more concerned with inequality than with health itself. The standard defence against the charge was, however, that health inequalities provided an important aetiological clue to the determinants of health. At least they served as an important reminder of the continued sensitivity of health to socio-economic factors. With what I thought at the time was a little wishful thinking I, like others, suggested that socio-economic differences in health might lead us to factors which had a crucial influence on the health of the whole population. I now feel rather taken aback to find that this is exactly what has happened. The results of a series of research projects – made possible by funding from the Economic and Social Research Council – suggest that the degree of socio-economic inequality in developed societies is a key determinant of the *average* standard of health of their populations. Figures 1 and 2 show clearly that, among the rich developed countries, it is not the richest countries which have the highest life expectancy, but the ones with the most egalitarian distribution of income.

As inequality has always been one of the central concerns of sociology these relationships place the determinants of health firmly in the sociological court. I would first like to go through the evidence which makes me think that the relationship between average life expectancy and income inequality is causal, and then go on to discuss some of the mechanisms which may be involved.

Income distribution and health: national and international evidence

The relationship between income distribution and health is quite robust. It has now been demonstrated several times on cross-sectional evidence, using different measures of income distribution, from different countries, at different dates (Rodgers 1979; Wilkinson 1986a and 1990; Le Grand 1987). More recently it has been shown that there is also a relationship between changes (over periods of five to ten years) in income distribution and in life expectancy in developed countries (Wilkinson 1992). As well as being robust, it is, in statistical terms, a strong relationship. Despite the small number of observations, the correlation coefficients are usually highly significant and suggest that as much as two-thirds of the variation in life expectancy between these countries may be related to the differences in their income distributions.

Table 1 Pearson correlation coefficients for relation between life expectancy (male and female at birth) and income distribution in nine countries in the OECD

		Everyone below each decile	
Income distribution	*Each interdecile group separately*		*Controlling for gross national product/head*
Decile 1	0.13	0.13	0.28
Decile 2	0.63*	0.45	0.57
Decile 3	0.76**	0.57*	0.66*
Decile 4	0.92***	0.65**	0.73*
Decile 5	0.64*	0.75**	0.83**
Decile 6	0.28	0.84***	0.91***
Decile 7	0.18	0.86***	0.90***
Decile 8	0.17	0.80**	0.81**
Decile 9	0.11	0.68*	0.68*
Decile 10	–0.68*		

*$p<0.05$; **$p<0.01$; ***$p<0.001$.

The best source of internationally comparable income distribution data comes from the Luxembourg Income Study. Table 1 is based on its figures for Australia, Canada, Netherlands, Norway, Sweden, Switzerland, (West) Germany, UK and USA in 1981 as published by Bishop *et al.* (1989). It

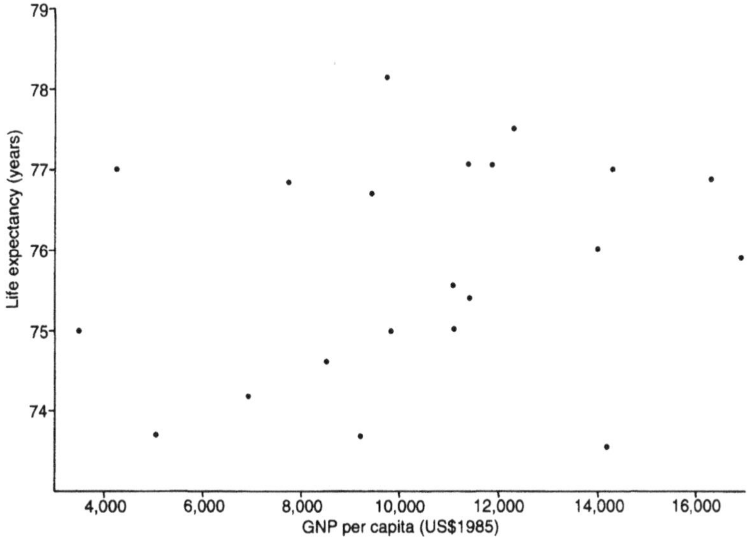

Figure 1 Relation between life expectancy at birth (male and female) and GNP per capita among OECD countries, 1985

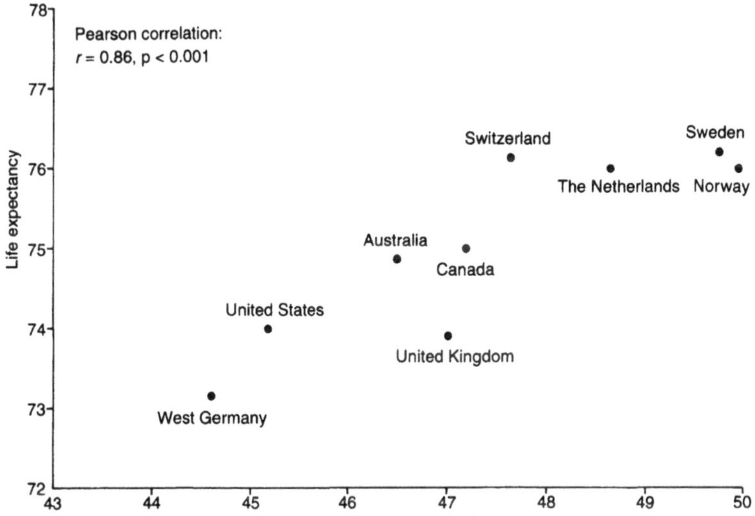

Figure 2 Relation between life expectancy at birth (male and female combined) and percentage of post tax and benefit income received by least well-off 70 per cent of families, 1981

shows the correlation coefficients between life expectancy at birth of males and females and the share of family disposable income (after taxes and benefits) received by various sections of the population. The first column shows the correlation between life expectancy in these countries and the share of income going to each successive tenth of the population, starting with the poorest tenth. Significant positive correlations are found over four out of five of the deciles in the lower half of the distribution and a negative correlation with the proportion of income going to the richest 10 per cent. All suggest that increased life expectancy is associated with a more egalitarian distribution of income. Instead of looking at each decile separately, column two shows the correlations between average life expectancy and the proportion of income received by the cumulated population below each successive decile. Thus the coefficient at decile 4, for example, is not just the correlation with the proportion of income going to the ten per cent of families in that decile but to the combined 40 per cent below that decile. Column 3 is on the same basis as column 2, but contains partial correlations controlling for Gross National Product per capita (at purchasing power parities). It is clear that controlling for GNP per capita makes little difference to the picture. The strength of the correlation with life expectancy builds up to a maximum at the share of income going to the bottom 60 or 70 per cent of the population. Figure 2 shows the association at the seventh decile in column 2. An equally strong cross sectional relationship has been shown using the Gini coefficient to measure income distribution in 1970 among a slightly different group of countries (Wilkinson 1986).

The intimate nature of this relationship becomes clear when we see that it holds between *changes* in life expectancy and income distribution over time. Comparable income distribution data is hard to find, but an attempt to measure changes in relative poverty (defined as those receiving less than 50 per cent of the average income) in European Community countries between 1975 and 1985 provided some useful figures (O'Higgins and Jenkins 1990). Figure 3 shows the relationship between changes in relative poverty and in the average life expectancy of people in each of the 12 European Community countries. Once again, the correlation is statistically significant and quite strong.

Figure 4 uses a third set of comparable data to take another look at changes over time. Using an OECD (1986) source it shows the relationship between the rate of changes in the share of income going to the least well-off 60 per cent of the population and the annual rate of increase in life expectancy. Once again, the countries whose income distribution has narrowed most rapidly (or widened most slowly) have experienced faster increases in life expectancy and, despite the small number of countries for which data are available, the relationship is strong enough to be statistically significant.

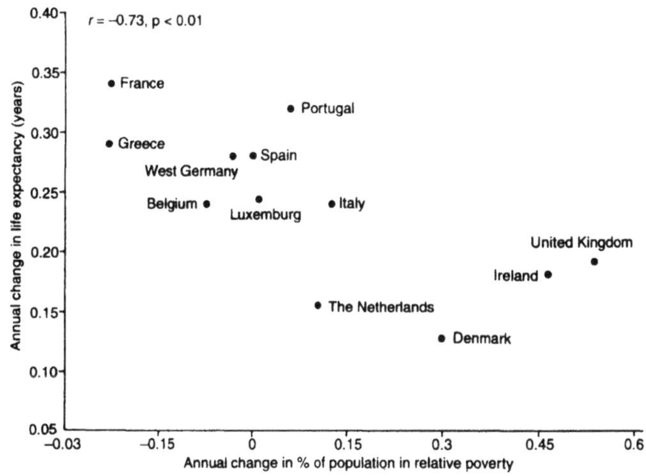

Figure 3 Annual rate of change in life expectancy and in proportion of population in relative poverty in 12 European Community countries, 1975–85

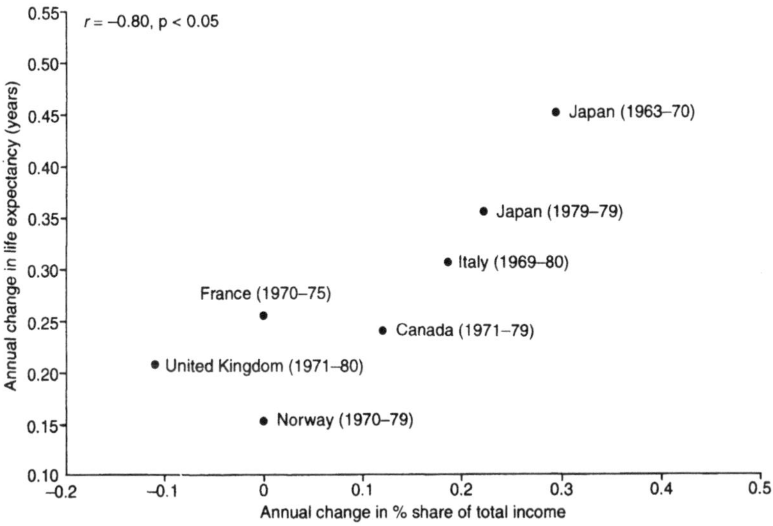

Note: Two figures for Japan were combined when calculating correlation coefficient.

Figure 4 Annual change in life expectancy and percentage of income received by least well-off 60 per cent of population

Some of the differences we are dealing with in income distribution may seem rather small, but they are associated with two- and three-fold differences in the proportion of people living in relative poverty and equally large differences in the ratio of incomes of those in the top and bottom 20 per cent of the income distribution. In addition, a difference of as little as four per cent in the share of income going to the bottom 70 per cent of recipients (say from 45 to 49 per cent as in Figure 1), means a four per cent decline in the share going to the richest 30 per cent, so that the effect on relative shares is doubled. If we also express this as a percentage change, not in the share of total *societal* income, but more meaningfully as the percentage change in the average income of people in the bottom 70 compared to those in the top 30 per cent, the original four per cent change becomes an improvement of over 17 per cent in the *relative* income of everyone in the bottom 70 per cent.

A less purely statistical picture of this relationship can be gained from the contrasting experience of Britain and Japan. In terms of both life expectancy and income distribution, the two countries were much like each other in 1970 and lay in the middle of the field of developed countries (Wilkinson 1986b). Since then Japan's income distribution has narrowed rapidly (see Figure 4) and it now has the most egalitarian income distribution in the developed world. Its life expectancy has improved equally dramatically to reach the highest recorded for any country (Marmot and Davey Smith 1989). In contrast, while Britain's income distribution worsened dramatically during the later 1980s to produce the largest inequalities in earnings for over a century, its position in the international life expectancy league table has also worsened. Mortality rates among both men and women between the ages of 15 and 44 actually rose throughout the late 1980s – a trend which the Chief Medical Officer pointed out was not attributable to the rise in deaths from AIDS (DHSS 1990).

Lest anyone think that Japanese progress is more a reflection of its rapid economic growth, it is worth emphasizing that the relationship in developed countries between life expectancy and GNP per capita is, at best, weak. Over the 16 years (1970–71 to 1986–87) among the 23 OECD countries, there was no significant relationship between changes in life expectancy and in GNP per capita (converted at purchasing power parities rather than at the less meaningful currency exchange rates). The correlation coefficient was 0.07 (Wilkinson 1992). (Any *cross-sectional* relationship with GNP per capita is covered by the partial correlation coefficients in the third column of Table 1 which control for GNP per capita.)

Time series evidence of an association between income differentials and life expectancy comes also from Winter's analysis of increases in life expectancy in Britain this century (Winter 1988). He pointed out that civilian life expectancy increased two or three times as fast during the two World Wars as it did during the rest of the century. Partly because of the virtual elimination of unemployment and partly because of trends in earnings, the two wars were periods of dramatic income redistribution (Wilkinson 1989). In addition both wars saw attempts to ensure the provision of at least minimum standards for all – a policy exemplified in the Second World War by food rationing. Although we are now used to emphasizing the health benefits of food rationing, it should not be forgotten that equally rapid gains in life expectancy occurred in the absence of food rationing during the First World War.

Reverse causation and intervening variables

Before going on to look at the ways in which income distribution might affect life expectancy, we should consider the possibilities of this relationship arising as a result of reverse causality or as an expression of some intervening variable associated with both income distribution and life expectancy. If sickness is sometimes the cause of poverty, a higher proportion of sick people would tend to widen the income distribution. Such processes of reverse causality have been carefully studied for their impact on class differences in health. Data from a number of longitudinal studies suggest that they make a fairly minor contribution to class differences in mortality (Power *et al.* 1990; Fox *et al.* 1990; Wilkinson 1986a). However, class differences are usually measured among economically active people of working age among whom these effects would be at their maximum. In contrast, the data used in the tables and figures shown above refer to life expectancy at birth of all people, whether economically active or not. The large proportion of the population who are children, pensioners or others who are not economically active will not suffer any loss of income when sick.

There is also an aspect of reverse causality which is likely to work in the opposite direction, tending to hide any causal effect income distribution may have on health. As life expectancy increases, a growing proportion of the population will be elderly. If, as is the case in most countries, the elderly are more likely to be poor, then a population with a long life expectancy may be expected to have a wider – rather than a narrower – income distribution. Indeed, there is some evidence that such an effect is detectable in data on life expectancy at older ages.

If we were, nevertheless, to disregard these factors and imagine that a wider income distribution was the result of poorer health standards, the closeness of the statistical association between these factors would imply that income distribution was largely determined by health. Economic factors such as taxes and benefits, profit levels, wage bargaining, unemployment etc. would be largely excluded. This implication would not wash with most economists. For these reasons I think we can dismiss the possibility that causality runs from improved life expectancy to a narrower income distribution.

The next consideration is that the relationship is an expression of some intervening variable related to both life expectancy and income distribution. We should note first that relationships as close as this are inherently less likely than weaker ones to result from intervening variables: the relationships with the intervening variable would have to be closer than the supposedly spurious relationship it gives rise to. But putting that aside for the moment, what are the possibilities?

The most plausible candidate might seem to be some area of public expenditure which benefits health. It seems likely that the provision of public services would be more extensive in more egalitarian societies. To assess the importance of factors of this kind I have used data for OECD countries taken from the United Nations *Human Development Report* (1991). Although only a few variables are available for all OECD countries, it is usually possible to look at the relationships among about 20 of them. On this data, the relationship between the various measures of mortality and total public expenditure is both insignificant and negative. This suggests that, if there is any relationship at all, it is not an association between higher public expenditure and higher life expectancy.

There was, however, a significant positive association between life expectancy and the proportion of public expenditure going to health and education combined. But there are reasons for not taking this at face value. These include the fact that the association was weaker, rather than stronger, than the association with income distribution, and was not supported by associations with other, more direct measures of educational and medical provision. Neither years of education nor total expenditure on education as a proportion of GNP played any significant role. Total health care expenditure as a proportion of GNP showed no sign of a relationship with mortality at all. This confirms Le Grand's (1987) finding on public and private expenditure on medical care. The relationship between life expectancy and the provision of doctors per head of population was *negative* and just reached statistical significance, implying that developed countries with higher life expectancy had fewer doctors per head. This curious association was first reported by Cochrane *et al.* in 1978 under the title 'The anomaly that would not go away'. Other evidence also suggests that medical services do not have a decisive influence on mortality in the developed world: even the small proportion of deaths from conditions regarded as wholly amenable to treatment seem less influenced by differences in medical provision than they are by differences in other socio-economic factors (Mackenbach *et al.* 1990).

If public services do not fit the bill, the only other possibility which has been suggested is that ethnic minorities may have poorer health and widen the income distribution as a result of discrimination in employment. The evidence suggests that ethnic minorities, at least in Britain, have very little effect on overall *national* standards of health (Balarajan and Bulusu 1990). One of the most impressive things about the effect we are dealing with here is (as we shall see below) that it is too large to be explained in terms of the health of any class or category of the population which does not constitute a majority of the population. Furthermore, the data in Figures 3 and 4 show changes in income distribution and life expectancy during periods when international migration, particularly of the unskilled, was only possible on a very small scale. Lastly, only if the health disadvantage of ethnic minorities was unrelated to their economic circumstances could any influence they have on the overall picture be properly regarded as contributing to a *spurious* association between income and health.

What factors one should consider as possible intervening variables depends partly on guessing what people of varying ideological persuasions might think plausible. Having run out of guesses I will turn to a discussion of evidence that relative income does indeed effect health in a way which might be expected to give rise to the observed international relationship. Most of this evidence comes from studies related to health inequalities in Britain.

Income and health within Britain

One would expect income differentials to have a bigger impact on the scale of socio-economic inequalities in health within each country than they do on the population's average mortality or life expectancy. When investigating the relationship between income and health differences, I found that the long-term trends in social class differentials in mortality in Britain appear to reflect trends in relative poverty (Wilkinson 1989). Class difference in death rates reached their narrowest on record in the early 1950s when relative poverty was reduced to an all time British minimum. Since then relative poverty has increased at an accelerating rate and mortality differences have widened decade by decade. Figures for the early 1980s, the latest available, showed mortality differentials were the widest recorded since accurate records began in 1921. (This statement is true even after allowing for the changing social class classification of the population and the changing proportion of the population in each social class.) Overall, while class difference in death rates moved from the narrowest to the widest on record, the same measure of relative income shows that the proportion of the population living in poverty increased from 6 per cent in 1953 to 23 per cent in 1983 (Piachaud 1988) and probably to about 30 per cent by the end of the 1980s. As Piachaud shows, only a very small part of this increase is attributable to the changing age-structure of the population: nearly all of it is a result of increases in poverty within each age group.

The most obvious explanation of the relationship between income distribution and life expectancy in developed nations is that there is a curvilinear relationship between income and mortality within each country such that income transfers from the rich to the poor benefit the health of the poor by more than they harm the health of the rich. A curve with this property was first shown using crude averages of income within each social class and were published in the OPCS Decennial Supplement on Occupational Mortality for 1971 (OPCS 1978). The most recent figures come from the Health and Lifestyles Survey (Blaxter 1990). The study used three different meas-

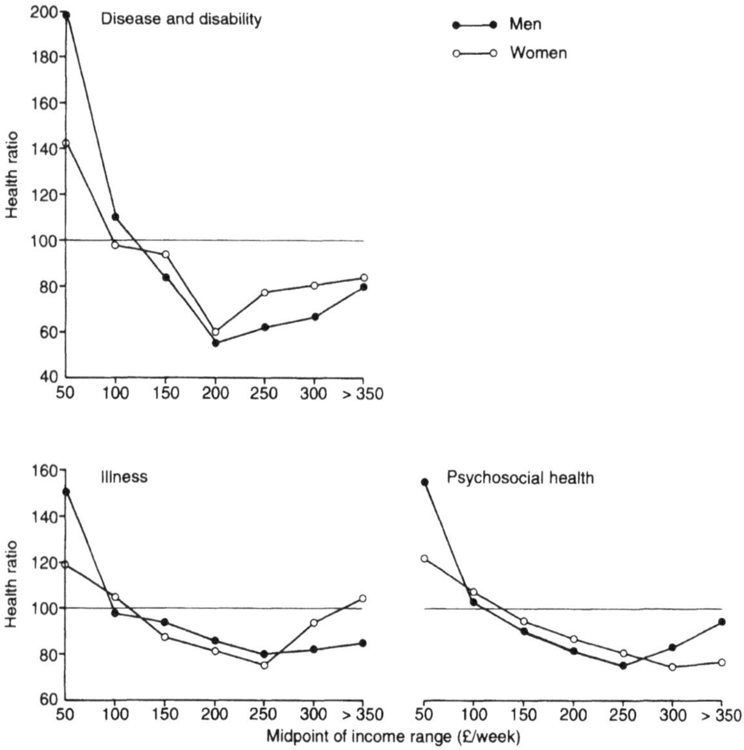

Figure 5 Age-standardized health ratios for disease and disability, illness and psychosocial health in relation to weekly income (£) in 1981, of men and women aged 40–59

ures of ill health and collected data from some 7,000 people in 1984 and 1985. The relationships found are shown in Figure 5. On each measure, health improves rapidly as you move from the lower towards the middle income categories. In addition, despite being confined to one age group, each measure suggests some deterioration in health at the higher income levels. If these cross-sectional relationships were even partly causal, they would suggest that income redistribution might have a dramatic effect on the health of the poor and may even benefit the health of the rich as well. The problem is to know whether they are causal or not.

A good test of causality is not easy to design. Though partly the beneficiaries and victims of circumstances, the rich and the poor are presumably also partly self-selected. Merely to control observations for differences in social class or education fails to deal with the host of more subtle differences that are likely to exist between people in different income groups. The same problems arise even if you record the health of people over time as they get richer or poorer. The only way round these problems is to examine the effects of income changes which are brought about by factors which are exogenous to the characteristics of the people affected. The most obvious opportunity to do this was simply to look at national death rates of old people in relation to the changing value of state old age pensions. As something like two-thirds of all old people live in relative poverty (DHSS 1979), one might expect an income effect on health to show up fairly clearly among them. Over a sixteen year period, I found a close relationship between the changing value of pensions and the death rates of old people (Wilkinson 1986b). The relationship held when I used GNP per capita to control for the effects of more general economic ups and downs, and it is also held when I controlled for changes in the death rates of middle aged people not yet old enough to receive pensions.

A more recent attempt to see whether health is responsive to changes in income involved analysing the relationship between changes during the decade 1971 to 1981 in the position of occupations in the earnings and mortality 'leagues' (Wilkinson 1990). Earnings data taken from the New Earnings Survey allowed changes in each occupation's mortality to be related to changes, not simply in its average earnings, but to changes in the distribution of earnings in each occupation. Highly significant correlations were found between changes in occupational mortality and changes in the proportion of relatively poor people in each occupation. Changes in each occupation's unemployment rate and in the proportion of people earning less than about 60 per cent of the national average were closely related to changes in occupational mortality rates.

These results were statistically significant and the data satisfied the requirements for using least squares regression. It is, of course, possible that more healthy people were selected into occupations as they went up the earnings league and vice versa. If so, one might expect the scale of this effect to be related to the size of the net flow of people in or out of an occupation. On this assumption, I used the percentage change in the size of each occupation to control for possible selective effects, but found it made no significant difference to results. It looks then as if there is an important effect of changes in income on health among the relative poor which probably peters out at average income levels. This in itself would lead one to expect income distribution and health to be related at the national level and was what led me, on Mildred Blaxter's advice, to look at the relationship between income distribution and mortality between countries.

Two characteristics of the explanatory problem

If the most plausible explanation of this relationship is that health is affected by relative income, the next question is what pathways, mechanisms or processes are responsible for the link?

When thinking about this problem, there are two points which should be mentioned at the outset. The first is that the scale of the effect of income distribution on health – indicated by the cross-sectional data – seems too large to be explained purely by a narrowing of socio-economic differences in health. A regression equation based on the data in Figure 1 suggests that if Britain were to adopt an income distribution more like the most egalitarian countries in Europe (not going as far as Japan), it would add about two years to average life expectancy. As social class V contains only about six per cent of the economically active population, reducing their death rates to the average would only add a few months to average life expectancy. To increase the average by two years would involve something like half the population overcoming a health disadvantage as great as social class V's. Because no group as large as this at such high risk has ever been identified (Goldblatt 1990), it suggests that the health effects of income distribution go beyond the reduction in class inequalities in mortality, at least as conventionally measured.

Two other considerations point in the same direction. While it is true that health inequalities between Japanese blue- and white-collar workers narrowed while that country's life expectancy improved so rapidly (Marmot and Davey Smith 1989), and Britain's class differences in death rates widened as income differentials widened, it is also clear that health inequalities have not been eliminated even in the most egalitarian countries. Although health inequalities seem to be smaller in more egalitarian countries such as Japan, Sweden and Norway, they nevertheless continue to exist (Fox 1989; Marmot and Davey Smith 1989). The implication is that the health benefits of an improved income distribution are not confined to the socially deprived or to any other minority.

The second factor which points in the same direction is the pattern of correlations in Table 1. Columns 2 and 3 suggest that health improves with the share of income going to the bottom 60 or 70 per cent of the population. Because income distribution is skewed by a few high earners, over 60 per cent of the population receive less than the average. It is therefore tempting to interpret the pattern of correlations in Table 1 as suggesting that the health of almost two-thirds of the population in receipt of less than average incomes may be improved by income redistribution.

The other general point which we need to bear in mind when thinking about mechanisms is that we are dealing with the effects of relative rather than absolute income. We saw earlier that the relationship between life expectancy and GNP per capita in developed countries is weak – whether you look at cross-sectional or longitudinal relationships. While this may seem puzzling, it becomes more understandable in the light of the relationship (Figure 6) between life expectancy and GNP per capita among both rich and poor countries. This suggests that below a certain level of income

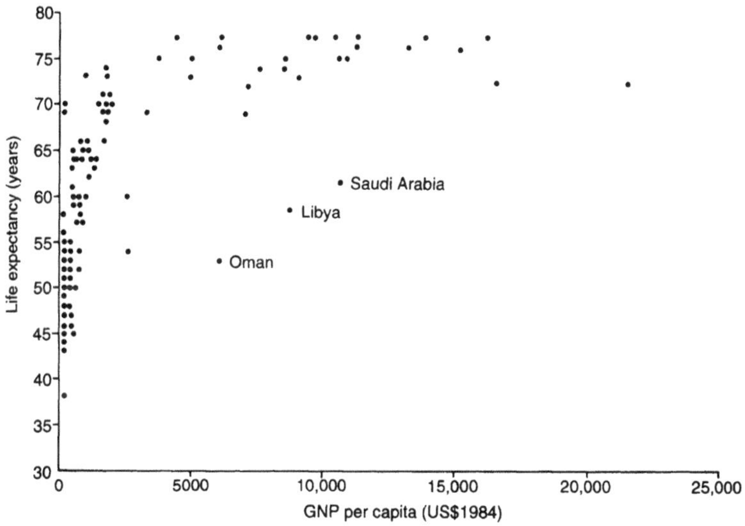

Figure 6 Relation between life expectancy at birth (male and female) and GNP per capita in rich and poor countries (with three named outliers)

the two are related, but once past this threshold level of absolute income, as all the developed countries are, the relationship peters out: average income levels can be as much as three times as high in some developed countries as in others without any appreciable gain in life expectancy. Unless income distribution generally worsens as countries get richer – which it does not – the amount of absolute poverty must be reduced by successive increases in GNP per capita. The lack of relationship between health and GNP per capita among these countries means that the health differences between them are not primarily a reflection of the extent of *absolute* poverty.

There are two additional reasons for thinking that we are not dealing with the effects of residual absolute poverty in the developed world. The first is simply that there are too few people in absolute poverty in each of the developed countries for their death rates to have a decisive influence on national death rates. The second is that while mortality rates are related to income distribution and to the proportion of the population in relative poverty, they are less obviously related to how poor the poor are (Smeeding *et al.* 1990:70). This, however, may well be a statistical artifact reflecting what looks like a tendency for the average degree of poverty among the poor to be greater in countries where fewer fall below the poverty line.

It looks, therefore, as if what matters to health in the developed world is no longer where we stand in terms of any absolute standards, but simply how we stand in relation to each other. Incomes and living standards appear to take on meaning and effect not directly in themselves, but in relation to standards elsewhere in society. If circumstances impact on health less of their own accord than through a comparative process, this suggests that psychosocially mediated effects may be crucial. To give an example, attempts to account for the ill health associated with damp housing in terms of the direct effects of dampness, have only been able to account for a very small part of the problem. While it was successfully demonstrated that the presence of mould spores in the air were responsible for some increase in rates of respiratory illness (Martin *et al.* 1987), most of the excess morbidity escapes this kind of analysis. If the link with relative poverty implies what I have suggested, then what people feel about their housing, their financial and social circumstances and what that does to their morale, is likely to be more important among most people than their objective conditions. This does not mean that there are not still substantial numbers of people in developed countries whose health is affected directly by absolute poverty. It means only that this is not central to the explanatory problem before us here.

Some possible mechanisms

Having just emphasized the importance of relative over absolute income and inferred that this indicates that psychosocial factors are likely to provide the crucial links with health, I should mention two possible pathways which either do not involve any social process of comparison or which may initially *appear* to result from an income which is inadequate in absolute rather than relative terms. The first is a function of the tendency for the *material* infrastructure and organization of society to be geared (by market forces) to people close to the average income. This means that people with lower incomes are often unable to equip themselves adequately to manage day to day tasks without a lot of additional effort. No doubt people's health will suffer to some degree simply as a result of the additional difficulty of coping with daily life. Even if other people's standard of living was invisible to them, their lives would be made objectively more difficult if other people's income increased faster than theirs. The most widely recognized (and overworked) example is that of people without cars being unable to benefit from supermarkets, having to shop at the more expensive remaining local corner shops and being cut-off from other activities by their dependence on a shrinking bus service. Another example might be the difficulty of managing without a washing-machine now that even council flats are equipped with plumbing for them and have sinks too small for washing by hand. Once, when there were still large numbers of households without washing-machines, local launderettes were an easy alternative; but as domestic machines have spread, they have become harder to find. One more example is the fact that most houses and flats are now build without a cool larder for food storage so that fridge-freezers are becoming a necessity – especially where employment stops people shopping daily.

The other apparent exception to the central role of psychosocial processes is the likelihood that incomes which may be adequate to provide for what are seen as the basic physiological necessities of an adequate diet, shelter, clothing and warmth etc., that is, to stave off absolute poverty, may not in practice be adequate to stave off what look like the effects of absolute poverty. The point here is only that people's social and psychological needs also have financial consequences: to keep body and soul together, an income must be adequate to maintain self-respect and to participate in the social life of a society where most people are much better off. Given the need to go out with friends occasionally, to have a television to relieve the boredom, or to buy your children clothes which don't disgrace you when parents gather at the school gates, incomes which may be adequate on paper to meet 'basic' needs may, in fact, mean people cannot afford a healthy diet and adequate heating. Hence small surveys have found that a quarter of all parents on what was then Supplementary Benefit had only one meal a day, and that at the end of the week a quarter of all people on unemployment benefit did not have enough money left for food (Burghes 1980; Lang *et al.* 1984). No doubt some of the seven per cent of pensioners which a DHSS (1979) survey found were malnourished had also failed to spend their pensions exclusively on 'necessities'. However, the inadequacy of the notional allowances for food and fuel used in the calculation of some benefits should not be forgotten (Stitt 1991).

I suspect that the practical visibility of these processes has sometimes led to them being emphasized at the expense of the less visible but more pervasive psychosocial costs of income differences. The processes we have mentioned may have an important effect on the health of a *minority* of the population: they must be important among the estimated 700,000 classified as homeless who live in bed-and-breakfast accommodation or worse (Greve and Currie 1990), and also among the 30 per cent or so of the population living in relative poverty. But the fact that the poor may skimp on food and warmth – for the sake of their self-esteem, social life or whatever – suggests that these problems are merely the symptoms of a deeper underlying social need whose satisfaction is made more difficult by income differences. Increasingly epidemiology is pointing to the influence on health of a wide range of psychosocial factors which might fit in here.

It is often assumed that most of the modern causes of death are understood better than they are. Lung cancer is one of the few important causes of death for which clearly identified risk factors account for most of the deaths. But if we look even at a disease as extensively researched as heart disease, we find that all major behavioural and physiological risk factors, whether potentially preventable or not, explain only about a third of the excess mortality in lower classes (Rose and Marmot 1981). In this situation there is a tendency to exaggerate the importance of the little that is known about prevention. The combined effect of the behavioural risk factors must account for a considerably smaller proportion of the excess risk in lower classes. For example, Rose (1981) using Framingham data, expressed the importance of a cholesterol lowering diet by saying that if, for forty years of their lives, men eat in such a way as to lower their blood cholesterol levels by 10 per cent, only 2 per cent would avoid a heart attack they would otherwise have had. In many other important causes of death our ignorance of causality is even greater.

Psychosocial factors

This lack of knowledge means that we can only make guesses as to the mechanisms which link mortality to income distribution. However, it looks as if the relationship with income distribution and the most promising lines of epidemiological research point in the same direction: namely, to psychosocial risk factors. Animal and human studies have suggested the involvement of immunological and hormonal pathways which could link psychosocial factors with a wide range of diseases (House *et al.* 1988; Madge and Marmot 1987). An increasing quantity of epidemiological research suggests that factors such as the extent and quality of people's social relations, stress and lack of control over work or one's circumstances may have important independent effects on mortality from a wide range of causes. 'Social support', 'confiding relationships', social participation have all been shown to be closely related to health (Berkman and Syme 1979; Cohen and Syme 1985; Brown and Harris 1978). The evidence suggests that the whole range of social relations have an influence on health – from the most personal domestic relations to relations at work, to people's participation in local community activities. After controlling for likely confounding factors, several well-conducted follow-up studies have shown that combined indices are predictive of two-fold differences in the all causes mortality rate (House *et al.* 1988).

Insofar as relative deprivation has been shown to be socially isolating (Townsend 1979), income differentials may affect social affiliations more widely. In the Whitehall Study of some 17,000 office-based civil servants, differences in social relations seem likely to play a part in explaining the three-fold difference in mortality between different occupational ranks. The most senior administrators were more likely to see a confidant daily, much more likely to have social contact with neighbours and much more likely to have social contact with people at work (Marmot 1986). But there are other possible links between social support and income: that disputes over money are a common cause of marital conflict presumably contributed to Brown and Harris's (1978) finding that women in lower social classes were less likely to have the benefit of a 'confiding relationship'.

There has been some controversy as to whether good social relations do more than protect against the health effects of stress (Cohen and Syme 1985). In contrast, there has been little or no work on the possibility that poor social relations, or contact across divisions of income, class, status etc. may actually be an important source of stress. There is, of course, a long tradition of regarding inequality as socially divisive at all levels in society. Though the experience of being 'up-staged' or 'put at a disadvantage' – which can intimidate and drain self-confidence – occurs at all levels in society, it must be a much more frequent experience lower down the hierarchy. Indeed, the loss of self-esteem and diminished sense of one's intelligence and abilities was one of the focal issues in Sennet and Cobb's (1973) study *The Hidden Injuries of Class*. To the extent that income and wealth are taken as indications of people's social status, of their importance and 'worth' as members of society, it seems likely that widening differentials will be psychologically harmful. Although relative poverty is widely understood to be a demeaning and devaluing experience, we tend to forget that it is only distinguished as a matter of degree from the sense of being of lesser worth which can spring from inequality almost anywhere in society.

The social organization of work is sometimes said to be the most important feature of occupational health for many employees. A cross-sectional study of 14,000 Swedish workers (men and women) found 'a more than multiplicative relationship' between the prevalence of cardiovascular disease and self-reported psychological job demands, people's degree of control over their work and the amount of social support they got from fellow workers (Johnson and Hall 1988). Disease was twice as common among people with high job demands, low control and low social support, even after controlling for other pertinent factors. There seems no reason why such a model should not operate in much the same way in the home environment. Just as increased pay differentials are likely to be associated with a deterioration in the psychosocial working environment, so inadequate relative incomes will increase stress, reduce people's ability to control their lives and make social contacts more difficult.

An additional link between income distribution and mortality may be provided by a number of behavioural risk factors. The use of tobacco and alcohol, and the taking of both prescribed and unprescribed drugs (which have collectively been referred to as 'drugs of solace' (Cameron and Jones 1985)), is often influenced by the quality of people's social relations and by factors such as stress and self-esteem. For example, several studies have shown that, despite the costs, people tend to smoke more when they become unemployed (OPCS 1984:194; Cook *et al.* 1982). However, data from the *UN Human Development Report* (1977) does not suggest that alcohol and tobacco consumption contribute to the international relationship between income distribution and life expectancy. Higher rates of crime and violence is another way in which widening income distribution may have psychosocial repercussions. As well as increasing levels of stress and insecurity, social participation among the elderly and others who feel vulnerable, may be curtailed by their fear of going out in the evenings.

Before leaving this subject, one additional angle on it should be mentioned. Although clear relationships between individual income and health have been found (see Figure 5), there have been suggestions that health is more closely related to what might be called 'financial stress' than to actual income (Calan *et al.* 1991; Ullah 1990). Even if there were only a weak relationship between individual relative income and health, the income distribution in a society could still have an important impact on health. Let us suppose, for example, that health is not actually the result of having a low relative income, but results from worries about money, from getting into debt, from not knowing whether you can pay for the next washing-machine repair or car insurance. One could hypothesize that there are people who are psychologically disposed to live up to the limits of their income and who always feel hard up even if their incomes are above the average. Similarly there are people with low incomes who clearly find them adequate enough not to have financial worries. If the tendency to buy more was a socially determined function of income distribution, (perhaps motivated by the need to maintain self-esteem), then a wider income distribution would mean that more people throughout society experienced financial stress. Although such an approach may seem attractive in a period when people are having houses repossessed because they cannot afford high mortgage interest rates, one would still expect financial stress to be fairly closely related to income.

Conclusions

The differences in health among the developed countries appear to be a psychosocially mediated function of income inequality. This raises theoretical and methodological problems which both epidemiologists and the medical profession are ill-equipped to deal with alone. Yet the issues are important and urgent. Although we are used to thinking of individuals as healthy or unhealthy, it looks as if we must think more in terms of healthy and unhealthy societies. Most of the suggestions we have discussed as to the ways in which income inequalities may affect overall standards of health have yet to be tested. But from the sociologists' point of view there is likely to be a two-fold interest in them. First is the issue simply of identifying the determinants of health as we have approached it here. Second, and equally interesting, is the possibility that we may simultaneously be learning about some of the major determinants of the quality of life. Health may serve as an indicator of the impact of various structural features on the subjective quality of life. As a measure of the quality of life, or of the real standard of living, income and other monetary indices suffer from an inability to get to grips with either qualitative (as opposed to quantitative) change or with the all-important psychosocial implications of the circumstances in which we live. As an alternative indicator of the quality of life, health may provide sociologists with an important additional source of hard data to bring to bear on some central issues of social organization.

Acknowledgements

I would like to thank: the British Medical Journal for permission to reproduce Table 1 and Figures 2, 3 and 4 from Wilkinson (1992); Routledge for permission to reproduce Figure 5 from Blaxter (1990); Polity Press for permission to reproduce Figure 6 from Marsh (1988); and the Economic and Social Research Council for financial support for a series of research projects on income and health.

References

Balarajan, R. and Bulusu, L. (1990), 'Mortality among immigrants in England and Wales 1979–83', in *Mortality and Geography: A Review in the mid-1980's, England and Wales*, London: Office of Population Censuses and Surveys, Series DS No. 9.

Berkman, L.F. and Syme, S.L. (1979), 'Social networks, host resistance and mortality: a nine year follow-up study of Almeda County residents', *American Journal of Epidemiology*, **109**:186–204.

Bishop, J.A., Formby, J.P., Smith, W.J. (1989), *International Comparisons of Income Inequality*, Luxembourg: Luxembourg Income Study, Working Paper 26.

Blaxter, M. (1990), *Health and Lifestyles*, London: Routledge.

Brown, G.W. and Harris, T. (1978), *Social Origins of Depression*, London: Tavistock.

Burghes, L. (1980), *Living from hand to mouth: a study of 65 families living on supplementary benefit*, London: Child Poverty Action Group and Family Service Unit.

Calan, T., Nolan, B. and Whelan, C.T. (1991), *Resources, Deprivation and the Measurement of Poverty*, Working Paper 21, The Economic and Social Research Institute, Dublin.

Cameron, D. and Jones, I.G. (1985), 'An epidemiological and sociological analysis of the use of alcohol, tobacco and other drugs of solace', *Community Medicine*, **7**:18–29.

Cochrane, A.L., St Leger, A.S. and Moore, F. (1978), 'The anomaly that would not go away', letter, *The Lancet*, 25 November.

Cohen, S. and Syme, S.L., (eds) (1985), *Social Support and Health*, London: Academic Press.

Cook, D.G., Cummings, R.O., Bartley, M.J. and Shaper, A.G. (1982), 'Health of unemployed middle-aged men in Great Britain', *Lancet*, **I**: 1290–4.

Department of Employment (annually) *New Earnings Survey*, London: HMSO.

DHSS (1979), *Nutrition and Health in Old Age*, Reports on Health and Social Subjects, No. 16, London: HMSO.

DHSS (1990), *On the State of the Public Health*, Annual Report of the Chief Medical Officer, London: HMSO.

Fox, A.J. (ed.) (1989), *Health Inequalities in European Countries*, Aldershot: Avebury.

Fox, J., Goldblatt, P., Jones, D. (1990), 'Social class mortality differentials: artifact, selection or life circumstances?', in Goldblatt, P. (ed.), *Longitudinal Study 1971–1981: Mortality and Social Organisation*, London: HMSO, OPCS series LS: No. 6.

Goldblatt, P. (1990), 'Mortality and alternative social classifications', in Goldblatt, P. (ed.), *Longitudinal Study 1971–1981: Mortality and Social Organisation*, London: HMSO, OPCS series LS: No. 6.

Greve, J. and Currie, E. (1990), *Homelessness in Britain*, Joseph Rowntree Memorial Trust.

House, J.S., Landis, K.R. and Umberson, D. (1988), 'Social relationships and health, *Science*, **241**:540–5.

Johnson, J.V. and Hall, E.M. (1988), 'Job strain, work place social support, and cardiovascular disease', *American Journal of Public Health*, **78**, (10): 1336–41.
Lang, T., Andrews, C., Bedale, C., Hannon, E. and Hulme, J. (1984), *Jam Tomorrow*, Food Policy Unit, Manchester Polytechnic.
Le Grand, J. (1987), 'Inequalities in health: some international comparisons, *European Economic Review*, **31**: 182–91.
Mackenbach, J.P., Bouvier Colle, M.H. and Jougla, E. (1990), 'Avoidable mortality and health services: a review of aggregate studies', *Journal of Epidemiology and Community Health*, 44:106–11.
Madge, N. and Marmot, M.G. (1987), 'Psychosocial factors in health', *Quarterly Journal of Social Affairs*, **3**, (2): 81–134.
Marmot, M.G., (1986), 'Social inequalities in mortality: the social environment', in Wilkinson, R.G. (ed.), *Class and Health: Research and Longitudinal Data*, London: Tavistock.
Marmot, M.G. and Davey Smith, G. (1989), 'Why are the Japanese living longer?' *British Medical Journal*, **299**:1547–51.
March, C. (1988), *Exploring Data*, Cambridge: Polity Press.
Martin, C.J., Platt, S.D. and Hunt, S.M. (1987), 'Housing conditions and illhealth', *British Medical Journal*, **294**:1125–7.
OECD (1986), *Living Conditions in OECD Countries: a compendium of social indicators*, Paris: OECD.
O'Higgins, M. and Jenkins, S.P. (1990), 'Poverty in the EC', in Teekens, R. and Van Praag, B.M.S. (eds), *Analysing Poverty in the European Community*, Luxembourg: EUROSTAT.
OPCS (1978), *Occupational Mortality 1970–2*, Decennial Supplement, HMSO.
OPCS (1984), *General Household Survey, 1982*, London: HMSO.
Piachaud D., (1988), 'Poverty in Britain 1899 to 1983', *Journal of Social Policy*, **17**,(3): 335–349.
Power, C., Manor, O., Fox, J. and Fogelman, K. (1990), 'Health in childhood and social inequalities in health in young adults', *Journal of the Royal Statistical Society*, **153**:17–28.
Rodgers, G.B., (1979), 'Income and inequality as determinants of mortality: an international cross-sectional analysis', *Population Studies*, **33**:343–51.
Rose, G. (1981), 'Strategy for prevention', *British Medical Journal*, **282**:1847–51.
Rose, G. and Marmot, M. (1981), 'Social class and coronary heart disease', *British Heart Journal*, **45**:13–19.
Sennett, R. and Cobb, J. (1973), *The Hidden Injuries of Class*, New York: Knopf.
Smeeding, T.M., O.'Higgins, M. and Rainwater, L. (1990), *Poverty, Inequality and Income Distribution in Comparative Perspective*, London: Harvester.
Stitt, S. (1991), 'Poor income/poor health' paper presented at the British Sociological Association Annual Conference, Manchester.
Townsend, P. (1979), *Poverty in the United Kingdom*, Harmondsworth: Penguin Books.
Ullah, P. (1990), 'The association between income, financial strain and psychological well-being among unemployed youths', *Journal of Occupational Psychology*, **63**:317–30.
United Nations (1991), *Human Development Report*, Oxford: Oxford University Press.

Wilkinson, R.G. (1986a), 'Socio-economic differences in mortality: interpreting the data on their size and trends', in Wilkinson, R.G. (ed.), *Class and Health: Research and Longitudinal Data*, London: Tavistock.
Wilkinson, R.G. (1986b), 'Income and mortality', in Wilkinson, R.G. (ed.), *Class and Health: Research and Longitudinal Data*, London: Tavistock.
Wilkinson, R.G. (1989), 'Class mortality differentials, income distribution and trends in poverty 1921–1981', *Journal of Social Policy*, **18**,(3): 307–35.
Wilkinson, R.G. (1990), 'Income distribution and mortality: a "natural" experiment', *Sociology of Health and Illness*, **12**,(4): 391–412.
Wilkinson, R.G. (1992), 'Income distribution and life expectancy', *British Medical Journal*, **304**:165–8.
Winter, J.M. (1988), 'Public health and the extension of life expectancy in England and Wales 1901–60', in Keynes, M. (ed.), *The Political Economy of Health and Welfare*, Cambridge: Cambridge University Press.

3 The gendered resource triangle: Health and resources in later life

Sara Arber and Jay Ginn

Introduction

It is ironic that research on inequalities in health largely neglects those age groups with the greatest ill-health and highest use of health resources, namely elderly people. It has also been predominantly concerned with inequalities in men's health. Latterly the inequalities in health literature has embraced inequalities in health among women (Moser *et al.* 1988; Arber 1990, 1991; Popay and Bartley 1989; Annandale and Hunt 1990), but the focus has been on women below statutory retirement age. In this chapter, we show for elderly people how the resource of physical health is linked with material resources and access to supportive care. These three key resources reinforce one another, and women are disadvantaged in all of them: the resource triangle is gendered.

Recent research has shown class inequalities in women's health are as strong as in men's (Arber 1989; 1990), and that women's health is related to their family circumstances as well as their position in the social structure (Arber 1991). Women with children living in disadvantaged material circumstances are most likely to have poor health. Popay and Bartley (1989) show how women's health is affected by their material circumstances as domestic workers. Similarly, research on inequalities in mortality rates among women has shown that women in disadvantaged circumstances, especially those living in local authority housing and without a car, have higher levels of mortality, in addition to the adverse effects of low social class (Moser *et al.* 1988). Payne (1991) provides a comprehensive review of research on inequalities in women's health, but does not mention older women.

This burgeoning of interest in inequalities in women's health has not extended to older women. More generally, inequalities among elderly people according to gender, class and race have been relatively neglected. The predominant assumption is ageist, that inequalities moderate in later life as biological age outweighs social factors in influencing health (Arber and Ginn 1991b). The omission of later life from the inequalities in health debate may reflect sexism as well as ageism, since women form two-thirds of elderly people, and the gender imbalance increases to three times more women than men above the age of 85 (Arber and Ginn 1991a).

Health is of central importance to the lives of elderly people. It is the key determinant of their ability to remain independent and autonomous. Physical health is the single most important factor predicting life satisfaction (Palmore and Kivett 1977), in contrast to those of younger age. For elderly women, health is the most frequently mentioned source of dissatisfaction and is their dominant concern in considering the future (Bearon 1989). Since health is of such pivotal importance, it is remarkable that socio-economic factors associated with good health in later life have been so little studied.

The Black Report (DHSS 1980) did not explicitly discuss inequalities in mortality or morbidity above the age of 65. Since then, research has examined class differences in the mortality of elderly men, but not of older women. Fox and his colleagues working on the OPCS Longitudinal Study have shown that working class men have higher mortality than middle class men aged 65–74 (Goldblatt 1990; Fox and Goldblatt 1982; Fox *et al.* 1983). The class gradients for men over 75 are comparable to those found at younger ages.

There is some British research on inequalities in morbidity among elderly people, which has examined previous occupational class. Taylor and Ford (1983; Taylor 1988) showed that working class elderly women and men had poorer health than their middle class counterparts, and Victor and Evandrou (1987; Victor 1989, 1991) found class differences in health based on the elderly person's last occupation. However, these studies have not examined other aspects of elderly people's lives which may have an impact on their health, such as current material disadvantage in terms of low income and poor housing.

A sociological analysis of inequality in health among elderly women and men needs to be premised on two understandings. First, elderly people need to be seen in terms of their biography; women's earlier roles in production and reproduction have profound implications for their well-being in later life. Second, elderly people's lives must be examined holistically. Much literature examines only one component part of elderly people's lives, for example their financial resources and poverty (Groves 1987) or their caring needs and how this constrains the lives of others (Nissel and Bonnerjea 1982). This chapter will provide a framework for understanding the interrelationship between health and other aspects of elderly women's and men's lives.

Our approach builds on a political economy perspective, in which inequalities of all kinds of resources – health, income, assets, access to informal and formal care – are seen as resulting from the power relations which structure society. The political economy of ageing (Estes *et al.* 1982; Estes 1984) focuses on the way the status and resources of elderly people are conditioned by their class position in the social structure, and by the overall socio-economic, political and cultural environment. This is not to suggest that elderly people are mere victims of the prevailing social structure; rather, that their situation results from the interplay of social constraints and their efforts to resist these. However, the political economy perspective needs to be reformulated with a feminist approach. We focus on how and why elderly women have fewer resources, and experience greater constraints on their lives than elderly men.

Independence and dependence: resources and constraints

A key concern of elderly people is to maintain independence and autonomy for as long as possible. 'The prospect of becoming dependent on others for basic needs is regarded with trepidation by most of us. Dependency in adulthood threatens cherished values of self-respect and human dignity' (Braithwaite 1990:1). Dependence suggests a relationship in which there is an unequal distribution of power, and a lack of alternatives. The question of 'dependency' has been central to a great deal of research and writing about elderly people, both at the societal and the individual level. However, there has been less attention to the ways in which the various forms of dependency are gendered and structured within society. Some kinds of dependency are more damaging to dignity and social status than others. The financial dependence of children, houseworker women, and elderly people on waged men or the state is socially visible and has negative connotations, resulting in reduced power and status. This contrasts with the dependence of employees on employers for jobs, and of men on women for domestic/caring services, which is rarely acknowledged as dependency and entails little if any loss of autonomy, status or power. If all people are dependent, some are more so than others, in terms of the subordinate status they acquire.

The meaning and effect of dependence becomes clearer if we distinguish the level at which it occurs, whether the individual is dependent on other household members, on relatives or friends, or on the state. We suggest that resources and constraints need to be conceptualized as operating at the level of the individual, and at three other levels: members of the individual's household; the community, encompassing friends, neighbours and family members beyond the household; and the state.

For elderly people, it is essential to distinguish three key types of resources and to examine how they interrelate. The absence of any one of these acts as a constraint on the well-being of the individual, increasing the likelihood of dependency. They are: first, the bodily resources of health and functional abilities of the individual and other household members; second, material or structural resources such as income, assets, car ownership, housing and the quality of the home environment; and third, access to personal, domestic and health care. These three sets of resources form an interlocking Resource Triangle, as shown in Figure 1. Structural characteristics of the individual, their gender, class and race, influence the likelihood of possessing each type of resource (Arber and Ginn 1991a).

This chapter examines the interrelationships of these three sets of resources showing how the resource triangle is gendered, with older women systematically disadvantaged in each of these three key resources.

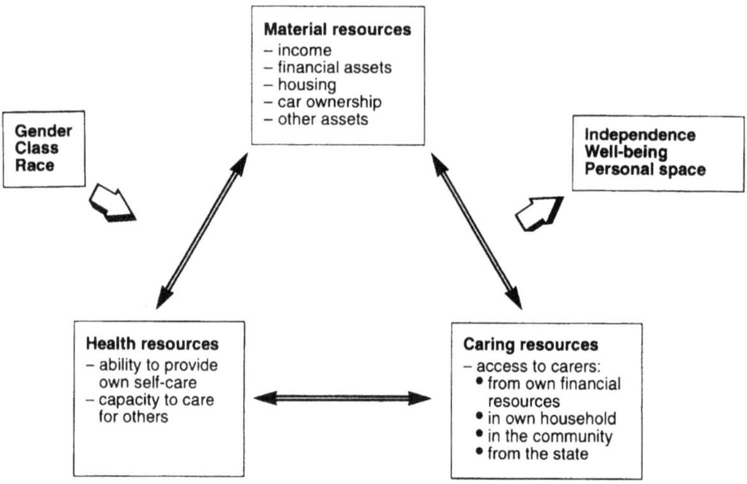

Figure 1 Three key resources influencing independence and dependence

Methods

Health, material and caring resources are examined using secondary analysis of national data from the British General Household Survey (GHS). The GHS is an annual interview survey of all adults aged over 16 in a representative sample of approximately 10,000 private households. It provides very high quality data, with a response rate of about 83 per cent (OPCS 1987). The survey yields data on about 4000 people over the age of 65 each year. We use data from the 1985 GHS for analyses of disability and caring, and data for 1985–87 for analyses of financial resources and self-assessed health.

Our measure of class is based on the elderly person's own last occupation. Occupations were categorized by the GHS into socio-economic groups, which we have collapsed into a five category class scale, with the addition of 'never worked' for the 16 per cent of elderly women who have never had paid employment.

Health and physical disability

Good health is essential to independence, especially the individual's capacity to carry out personal self-care, such as bathing, eating, negotiating stairs and walking outside the home. Chronic illness and disability tend to restrict the individual's independence, as well as generating extra costs for a special diet, additional heating, laundry, or nursing care. Those with higher levels of functional disability or cognitive impairment will require more practical support and personal care from either informal carers or the state. Since disability and good health are so essential to the maintenance of independence, it is pertinent to examine gender and class differences in personal health resources. The GHS provides no measures of the mental health of elderly people.

Our discussion of health is restricted to two measures of health included in the GHS, self-assessed health and functional disability. Self-assessed health has been found to be closely allied to feelings of well-being and quality of life (Hughes 1990). Poor self-assessed health is important to study because of its association with early mortality (Welin *et al.* 1985; Mossey and Shapiro 1982; Singer *et al.* 1976) and with institutionalization, after controlling for age and other health variables (Shapiro and Tate 1988).

Gender differences in self-assessed health are relatively modest in later life and are less important than differences associated with class. Respondents in the GHS were asked whether their health had 'on the whole been good, fairly good or not good' over the last year. About five per cent more women than men assess their health as 'not good' in each age group.

Figure 2 shows a strong social class gradient for self-assessed health for both elderly men and women. At least twenty per cent more 'higher mid-

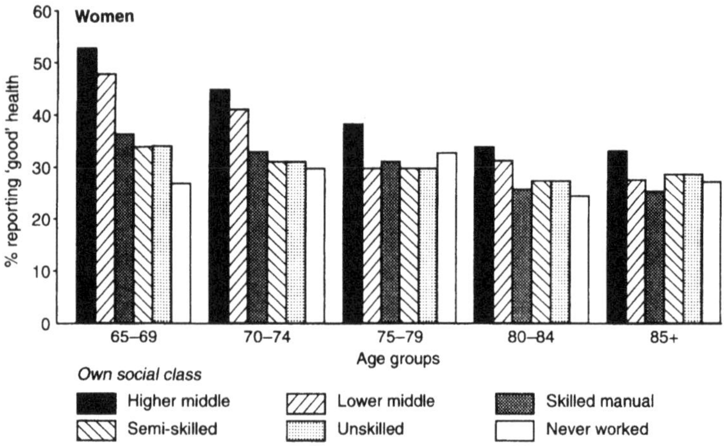

Source: General Household Survey, 1985–87 (authors' analysis).

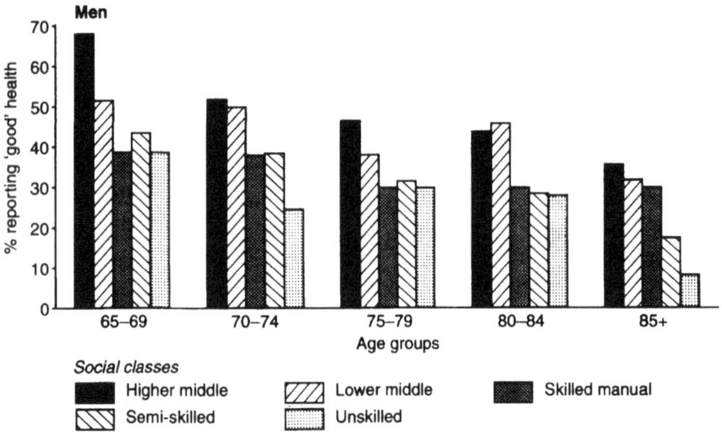

Source: General Household Survey, 1985–87 (authors' analysis).

Figure 2 Percentages of men and women reporting 'good' health by social class and five year age groups

dle' class men assess their health as 'good' compared to unskilled men within each age group. The class differential is almost thirty per cent among the 65–74 age group, and is still maintained among those aged over 85, where a third of 'higher middle' class men, compared to only eight per cent of previously unskilled men, rate their health as 'good'. For elderly women, the class differences are strongest among those in their late sixties. Elderly women who have never worked report poorer health than other women.

It may be considered surprising that such strong class gradients are found, given that for elderly people occupational class is based on their labour market position many years earlier, especially for women of this generation who may not have worked since marriage.

Another indicator of material circumstances is current income. Any measure of income needs to take into account the size of the elderly person's household and the relationships within the household. Since we cannot assume that income is equally divided between all household members when elderly people share a household with younger kin, our analyses exclude this minority, and are restricted to elderly people who either live alone or share a household with one other elderly person. (These will usually be married couples.)

Elderly people at the higher end of the income distribution, that is the top ten per cent in income, are substantially more likely to report good health than other elderly people (Table 1). The sharpest gradient is for married men aged 65–74 where 69 per cent of the top income decile report good health, compared with under a quarter of the lowest decile. For married women of the same age, there is a comparable income gradient in reporting good health from two-thirds of the highest decile, to under a third of the lowest thirty per cent. For married women aged over 75, self-assessed health is poorer, but the income gradient is similar, half of the top decile report good health compared with less than a fifth of the poorest thirty per cent.

For elderly people living alone, there is a clear advantage in self-assessed health for those with incomes in the highest thirty per cent, but little difference among other income categories. This lack of differentiation is largely because there is little variation in the income levels of elderly women who live alone and lone elderly men above 75, since these people are almost entirely reliant on the state pension.

Research reported elsewhere (Arber and Ginn 1993) shows that both occupational class, based on previous labour market position, and current income have statistically significant independent effects on the subjective health of elderly women and men. Therefore, in spite of elderly people having left the labour market a number of years earlier, higher occupational class continues to be associated with better self-assessed health.

Table 1 Percentage assessing their health as 'good' by income deciles: (a) for elderly men and women living alone; (b) for elderly men and women sharing their household with another elderly person

	Lowest decile	10%< 30%	30%< 50%	50%< 70%	70%< 90%	Highest decile	All
(a) Elderly person lives alone							
Men							
65–74	(35)*	33	31	48	47	56	45
75+	30	34	31	33	38	48	36
Women							
65–74	36	29	31	33	44	53	37
75–84	38	24	26	27	34	52	29
85+	27	24	30	32	43	(50)*	31
(b) Two elderly person household							
Men							
65–74	24	39	40	38	52	69	44
75+	24	24	33	39	45	50	33
Women							
65–74	30	27	34	42	50	67	41
75+	20	17	35	32	34	49	29

*Base number below 20.

Source: General Household Survey, 1985–87 (authors' analysis).

Current income has an additional effect in contributing to better subjective health.

Level of functional disability was measured using six items from the 1985 GHS. These included three questions about the elderly person's ability to perform tasks of personal self-care – washing/bathing, cutting their toenails, and getting into and out of bed; and three questions on aspects of mobility – walking down the road unaided, getting up and down stairs, and ability to get around the house. Each of these six tasks was divided into (0) could be done easily by the elderly person unaided, (1) could only be done with difficulty, and (2) could not be done unaided. The six items were

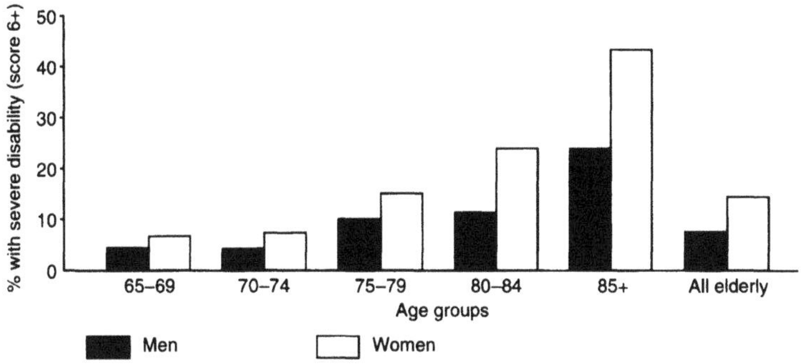

Source: General Household Survey, 1985 (authors' analysis).

Figure 3 Percentage with severe disability by sex and five year age groups

summed to form a scale which ranged from zero to 12. They formed a Guttman scale. (For details see Arber and Ginn 1991a.)

Elderly women are more likely than elderly men to be substantially disabled, and the gender difference increases with advancing age (Figure 3). Twice as many elderly women as elderly men have a severe level of disability (a score of six or more), 14 per cent compared with seven per cent. Elderly people with severe disability will have difficulty washing/bathing unaided and will be unable to walk down the road unaided. This level of disability is likely to require some provision of domestic and/or personal care/support on a regular basis. Gender differences are particularly striking at the oldest ages; a quarter of women aged 80–84 have severe disability compared with 11 per cent of men, and above the age of 85, 45 per cent of elderly women, compared with under a quarter of elderly men, are severely disabled. Thus elderly women are disadvantaged compared to men of an equivalent age, since they will require a good deal more care and support, simply to accomplish the activities of daily living.

Disability is not only gendered, but is structured by social class. Men and women who were previously in semi-skilled and unskilled occupations have a higher level of disability (Arber and Ginn 1991a; 1993). Despite the imprecision of measuring social class according to the individual's own last occupation, especially for elderly women who may not have been in paid employment for many years, class still reveals substantial inequalities in disability, as well as in self-assessed health. However, in Arber and Ginn (1993) we show that, unlike subjective health, disability is not associated with current income independently of class.

There are interconnections between types of resources. An individual with greater material resources is likely to be in better health; whilst, a cold, damp home and inadequate diet, due to poverty, jeopardize health. But if a person does become functionally disabled, financial resources help to offset the effects. A high income enables aids and adaptations to be obtained which facilitate independent living and the maintenance of personal autonomy, while extra costs of heating, laundry, or a special diet can be met without sacrificing other necessities.

Material resources and dependence

For women of all ages, the basis of their material disadvantage is the social expectation of their financial dependence on men within marriage. Women's generally lower pay, together with the constraints on participation in paid work placed on those who perform a reproductive role, has profound implications for women in later life, especially following widowhood or divorce. Thus dependencies established at an earlier stage of the life course impact on the individual's ability to remain independent in later life. Personal income, or money over which the individual has direct command, is a primary source of independence, enabling the individual to express their own priorities in meeting their physical and social needs.

The GHS data show that elderly women have a lower personal income than elderly men, see Figure 4. The state's role in providing financial resources to elderly people is largely an equalizing one, see first pair of boxplots. The middle 50 per cent of elderly men all receive between £38 and £43 from the state each week. For women there is more variation, from £23 to £40 (£23 representing the amount received in 1985 by a married woman dependent on her husband's contributions – the Wife's Allowance). The median level of state income for women, £37, is only slightly less than that for men, £40.

The second pair of boxplots shows the distribution of income from occupational and private pensions, for the 64 per cent of men but only 27 per cent of women who receive such income. The spread of non-state pension income for elderly men is very wide, the middle 50 per cent receiving between £8 and £43. Elderly women's pension income distribution is both lower and more compressed, with the middle 50 per cent receiving between £7 and £25. The median for men is £20, and for women £13.

Total personal income (third pair of boxplots), includes income from the state, from non-state pensions, from earnings, and from all other sources of regular income. The median for elderly men is £55 per week, and the

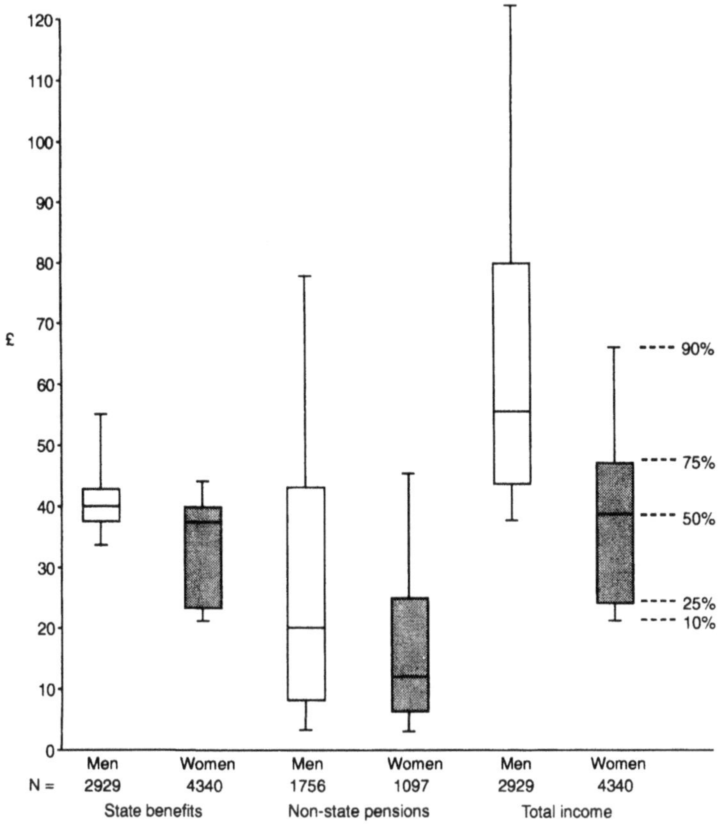

Source: General Household Survey, 1985–86 (authors' analysis).

Figure 4 Distribution of personal income from different sources in £ per week, elderly men and women

amount received by the top 25 per cent (upper quartile) is £80 per week. Elderly women's income falls far below men's, with a median of £39 – only two pounds higher than that received from the state – and an upper quartile amount of £46. The major reason for the gender difference in total income arises from women's lesser entitlement to occupational and private pensions. This reflects gender differences in the labour market and in employment histories during the 'working life' (Ginn and Arber 1991).

Class position in the labour market during adult life has a major impact on the financial well-being of elderly people. The likelihood of receiving an occupational or private pension is strongly associated with higher socio-economic status, and the gender difference holds within each class (Ginn and Arber 1991). Thus the availability of financial resources to facilitate autonomy and independent living in later life is critically linked to gender and social class.

Gender is associated with inequality in other material resources, such as housing and car ownership. Elderly men are more likely to be home owners than elderly women, 53 per cent compared with 48 per cent (GHS, 1985 authors' analysis). Over half of elderly men have a car in their household, which is 20 per cent higher than for women, although the gender differential declines among those over 80 years of age (Arber and Ginn 1991a). However, the gender difference in opportunity to benefit from a car in the household is likely to be even greater, since women are less likely to hold a driving licence, and have independent use of the car (Dale 1986). Elderly women's limited access to a private car is particularly restricting, since as we have shown they are more likely than men to have impaired mobility, and they are more likely to fear attack when walking in the street, or when waiting for buses and trains.

Elderly people with a higher occupational class are advantaged in home ownership, possession of consumer durables and other goods (Evandrou and Victor 1989), as well as in income. Thus gender and class affect the likelihood of possessing the material resources which allow greater comfort, freedom and independence in later life. But the constraints on autonomy due to lack of material resources are magnified when combined with structured inequalities in health.

A high degree of independence, due to possession of material and health resources, is generally accompanied by psychological well-being. Atchley (1982) finds a strong association for elderly people between a high level of leisure activities and life satisfaction. Both these outcomes depend on the same enabling conditions, especially good health and an adequate income. The implication is that lack of income inhibits the social and other activities which maintain normal functioning and enjoyment of life.

Access to caring resources and dependence

Poor health and disability may have profound implications for the elderly person's self-image and self-esteem. Women's higher level of disability makes them more vulnerable to such penalties of ageing. However, the likelihood of a given level of disability having these effects depends on the nature and availability of caring resources as well as on material resources.

Gender is associated with the nature of care provided to elderly people in two ways: (a) in terms of the kin relationship between the care-giver and care-receiver; and (b) whether care is provided within the household, by the community or by the state. We argue that the source of care, whether from a member of the household, the community or the state, has implications for the elderly person's sense of autonomy and self-identity. Elderly women are disadvantaged in terms of both the lack of closeness of their relationship to the carer and the setting in which care is provided.

Elderly women live on average for six more years than men (CSO 1989, Table 7.2). A consequence of women's mortality advantage, and of the cultural expectation that women marry men who are older than themselves, is that a much higher proportion of elderly women than men are widowed. Differential rates of widowhood are reflected in gender differences in living arrangements. Table 2 shows that half of all elderly women live alone, compared with a fifth of elderly men. Only 36 per cent of elderly women live with their spouse compared with seventy per cent of elderly men.

Table 2 Living arrangements of elderly men and women (column percentages)

		All elderly people		Severely disabled* elderly people	
		Men	*Women*	*Men*	*Women*
Living alone		20	48	21	43
Living in own household	– with spouse	70	36	63	30
	– with others (mainly adult children)	6	8	8	12
Living in another's household	– with adult children	2	5	6	12
	– with others	2	3	2	3
Total		100%	100%	100%	100%
N =		1477	2155	107	302

*Disability score over 6.

Source: General Household Survey, 1985 (authors' analysis).

The seven per cent of elderly women and 14 per cent of elderly men with severe functional disability need help with activities of daily living or personal self-care on a daily basis. Table 2 shows that among the severely disabled, 43 per cent of elderly women live alone compared with a fifth of elderly men. Thus, among elderly severely disabled people, women are twice as likely as men to live alone and therefore to be reliant on family members living elsewhere, other informal carers in the community, and state provided domiciliary services. This contrasts with the majority of severely disabled elderly men who can rely on support and care provided by their wife. Severely disabled elderly women are twice as likely as equivalent men to live in the home of an adult child (12 per cent) or to share their own household with other people (12 per cent), such as their unmarried children or siblings.

Care from the state, from family members or from a range of different providers in the community should not be treated as equally acceptable from the point of view of the care-receiver. The nature of that provision and the extent to which individuals perceive themselves as dependent is affected by the source of care, especially for personal care. Care provided by a spouse is the form of care generally preferred by the elderly person, and is less likely to be perceived by both partners as interfering with other aspects of the care-giver's life (Arber and Ginn 1992). This contrasts with care provided by a married daughter, where the care-giver is more likely to feel constrained and the elderly person more likely to be perceived as, and to feel, a burden. Because of elderly women's higher likelihood of being widowed and their greater disability, this potentially uncomfortable situation is experienced more often by elderly women than men.

The providers of care to an elderly person can be divided into six categories: (i) a marital partner, (ii) another household member, usually an adult child, (iii) a relative living elsewhere, usually a married daughter, (iv) the community – friends or neighbours, (v) the state – domiciliary health and welfare services, and (vi) the individual's (or their family member's) own financial resources – paid care. Tables 3 and 4 summarize the extent to which personal care and domestic support are provided from each of these sources to severely disabled elderly women and men, for those living alone, elderly married couples and all elderly people. Where elderly people in the 1985 GHS said they could not perform various personal and domestic tasks, or only with difficulty, they were asked who helps them or performs these tasks. For each task, up to three helpers could be named. The total number of people mentioned was summed up separately for the personal tasks and the domestic tasks, and categorized into the above six groups of possible providers. The total number of sources of help are given at the base of the columns in Tables 3 and 4. The proportion of help provided by each of the six categories of carer is shown in the body of these tables.

Table 3 Proportion of help provided with personal care tasks by different carers to elderly men and women with severe disability, by living arrangements

		Lives alone			Married couple			All	All
		Men	*Women*	*All*	*Men*	*Women*	*All*	**Men***	**Women***
A	**Co-resident care:**								
(i)	By spouse	–	–	–	88%	85%	86%	66%	28%
(ii)	By adult child or other in household	–	–	–	3%	4%	4%	12%	32%
B	**Care from outside the household:**								
(iii)	Other relative	38%	53%	53%	3%	5%	4%	8%	20%
(iv)	Friend/neighbour	–	16%	14%	1%	1%	1%	1%	5%
(v)	Formal services	50%	29%	32%	5%	7%	6%	12%	14%
(vi)	Paid care	12%	1%	2%	–	–	–	1%	–
		100%	100%	100%	100%	100%	100%	100%	100%
Average number of sources of help		.78	1.01	.97	1.85	1.53	1.67	1.62	1.40
N =		(23)	(131)	(154)	(68)	(88)	(156)	(107)	(302)

Note: Personal care tasks were climbing stairs, feeding, getting to the toilet, shaving/brushing hair, bathing, washing face/hands, walking indoors

*Includes elderly people living in other types of household.

Source: General Household Survey, 1985 (authors' analysis).

Table 4 Proportion of help provided with domestic tasks by different carers to elderly men and women with severe disability, by living arrangements

		Lives alone			Married couple			All	All
		Men	*Women*	*All*	*Men*	*Women*	*All*	Men*	Women*
A	**Co-resident care:**								
(i)	By spouse	–	–	–	95%	76%	86%	65%	20%
(ii)	By adult child or other in household	–	–	–	–	2%	1%	14%	36%
B	**Care from outside the household:**								
(iii)	Other relative	39%	47%	46%	1%	9%	5%	9%	20%
(iv)	Friend/neighbour	11%	12%	12%	–	2%	1%	2%	5%
(v)	Formal services	40%	38%	38%	3%	8%	5%	9%	16%
(vi)	Paid care	8%	3%	4%	–	3%	1%	2%	2%
		100%	100%	100%	100%	100%	100%	100%	100%
Average number of sources of help		2.7	2.53	2.55	3.51	2.56	2.97	3.40	2.96
N =		(23)	(131)	(154)	(68)	(88)	(156)	(107)	(302)

Note: Domestic care tasks were shopping, sweeping floors, washing laundry and cooking
*Includes elderly people living in other types of household.

Source: General Household Survey, 1985, (authors' analysis).

Elderly men on average receive almost two-thirds of their personal and domestic care from their spouse (final two columns of Tables 3 and 4). This contrasts with elderly women who receive only 28 per cent of their personal care and a fifth of their domestic support from their spouse. The largest proportion of support for elderly women, about a third, is from others living in the same household, mainly adult children. A fifth is provided by relatives living elsewhere, mainly married daughters. Women receive more domestic support than men from the state, but there is little overall gender difference in the proportion of personal care received from the state. Thus elderly disabled women are more heavily dependent than elderly men on the state, relatives living elsewhere, and on friends and neighbours in the community, whose care may be less reliable. These overall gender differences are largely explained by the differential living arrangements of elderly women and men.

For elderly married couples, where one partner requires personal care, this is almost all provided by their spouse whether of not the carer is the husband or the wife (Table 3). This contrasts with domestic care (Table 4), where disabled husbands not only receive a good deal more domestic care (average number of sources of help – 3.5) than disabled elderly wives (average – 2.56), but wives provide all except five per cent of the domestic support for their disabled husbands, compared with husbands who provide 76 per cent of the domestic care for their wives. Disabled elderly wives receive more domestic care from relatives living elsewhere and from formal services.

Among elderly disabled people living alone, elderly men receive less personal care support than women living alone (on average 0.78 sources of help compared with 1.01), but slightly more domestic care support (2.7 sources of help compared with 2.53). Lone elderly disabled men receive proportionately more personal care from the state than equivalent women, which compensates for the lack of personal care provided by friends and neighbours and the lesser amount provided by relatives living elsewhere. Elderly disabled men living alone are the only group with any paid personal care – this may reflect both their greater financial resources enabling them to purchase such care, as well as cultural taboos against cross-gender provision of personal care (Ungerson 1983). The latter may be the main reason for the lack of personal care provision to elderly men by friends and neighbours. Frail elderly men who live alone are a particularly vulnerable group, who may need more state personal care to enable them to remain in the community.

Caring must be conceptualized as having two sides. The care-receiver may feel dependent and lack autonomy, and the care-giver may feel burdened by providing care. The provision of informal care to support others, whether in the same household or living elsewhere, places some limitations on the carer's life. Women in their forties and fifties may be still caring for their own children and in addition be called upon to care for their parents or parents-in-law. Brody (1981; 1985) has coined the phrase 'women in the middle' to describe the situation faced by such women who have multiple and often conflicting caring responsibilities. Women are more likely to be constrained by the obligations to provide informal care than men of the same age, and are likely to have little state support, especially where women are caring for a disabled elderly person living in the same household.

The greatest constraint on the lives of elderly people is generally considered to be giving up their own home and residing in a communal establishment, such as a nursing home or Local Authority Part III accommodation. This is the biggest fear of elderly people and a major concern of their relatives, that they should not be 'put away' (Finch 1989). The state is concerned about the level of institutional residence of elderly people because of the costs of such care to the Exchequer. Indeed, this has been the

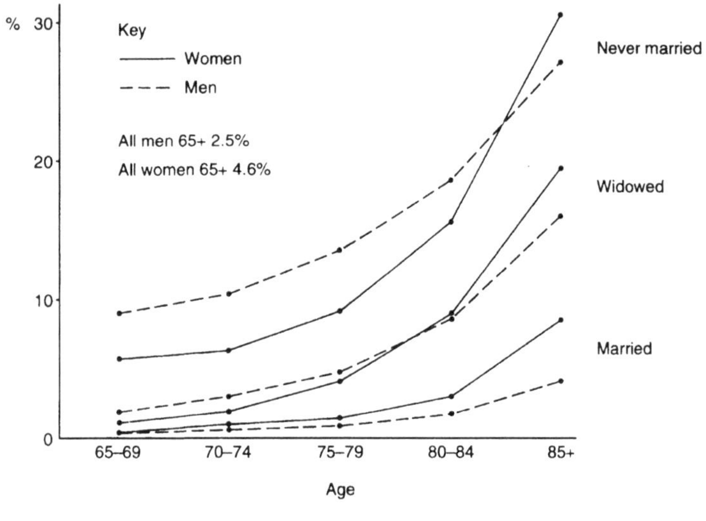

Source: OPCS (1984) *Census 1981, Communal Establishments, Great Britain*, London: HMSO, Table 5.

Figure 5 Percentage of elderly men and women resident in communal establishments by age and marital status, Britain 1981

main impetus of government policy in recent years, articulated as an aim to increase the 'caring capacity of the community' and reduce the use of institutional care (Department of Health 1989).

Figure 5 shows the percentage of elderly men and women in each marital status who were resident in a communal establishment at the time of the 1981 population census. The chances of institutional residence are closely related to marital status in each age group; married elderly people are least likely to be in residential care. For example, among elderly men in their late seventies, under one per cent of married men are in residential care, compared to five per cent of widowed men, and fourteen per cent of bachelors. The differences are somewhat smaller by marital status for elderly women, but still show an eight times higher rate of institutionalization among spinsters in their late seventies, compared with married women of the same age. These massive differences by marital status reveal the levels of informal care which are routinely provided, particularly by a spouse to their marital partner, but also by adult children (primarily daughters) to their widowed parents. The association between residential care and marital status, shows that those 'closest' to marriage and children are apparently most protected from institutionalization.

Comparing elderly men and women overall, the latter are nearly twice as likely to be in a residential setting, 4.6 per cent of elderly women compared to 2.5 per cent of elderly men. The main reason for this gender inequality is the greater chance of elderly women being widowed and living alone. This reflects women's greater longevity and the cultural norm that men marry a younger wife, as well as higher levels of remarriage for widowers than widows. For unmarried elderly people under the age of 85, the rate of institutionalization is higher for men than for women. This may reflect both the gender norm that sole elderly men are less able to provide their own domestic care and the lesser cultural acceptability of friends, volunteers and relatives providing personal care for elderly men who live alone, because of cross-gender taboos. Among married elderly people, it is only those few married elderly women over 75 years old who are more likely to be in residential care than married men of the same age.

Provision of resources – by the individual, family, community or society?

We will now look more closely at the various levels at which the three key resources can be provided and the implications of reliance on providers from particular levels. By outlining each level of provision in turn, we aim to assess the consequences for elderly women and men of reliance on different levels for the provision of resources. A schematic presentation of the four levels, indicating the nature of the key resources at each one, is given in Figure 6.

		Resources	
Levels	*Material*	*Health*	*Caring*
Individual	Income Housing Car Other assets	Own health	Ability to care for oneself Ability to care for others
Co-resident family members (The household)	Income Housing Car Other assets	Health of others in household	Willingness and ability of others in household to provide care
The community (relatives, neighbours, friends, volunteers)	Affluence of area (social class composition) Cultural norms of reciprocity	Health status of the community	Willingness of relatives, friends, and neighbours to provide care
The state	Pensions Income support Housing Public transport Public safety	Health care – GPs – hospitals – nursing homes	Domiciliary support – Home helps – Aids/adaptation – Meals on wheels – Community nurses

Figure 6 Availability of resources at four levels

The personal level A major resource of individuals is their own health, and thus their ability to look after themselves (personal self-care). Where disability makes this impossible, the individual is constrained, and is likely to become dependent on others for help with personal tasks, entailing loss of fully adult status. We have shown how health in later life is closely associated with position in the labour market during adult life, those previously in manual occupations having the highest levels of physical disability and poorer self-assessed health. Although women live longer than men, they suffer higher levels of disability and therefore have a greater need for care in later life.

Few individuals in the mid 1980s paid for their own personal care or domestic service provision, other than a small proportion of elderly men who lived alone. Given the individualistic focus of present British government policies, it is pertinent to consider how realistic it is to require elderly individuals to provide financial resources to support themselves. The capacity to do so is socially structured; women are disadvantaged compared to men, and those in more favourable positions in the labour market will be better able to provide occupational or personal pensions for themselves in later life than those who have been in worse positions. Those who have spent longer outside the paid labour force will be least able to manage without state support.

The household – co-resident family members State policies and benefit regulations are founded on the assumption that married women have claims to economic support from their husbands (Land 1989) and that resources within a co-resident family are equally shared among family members (Land 1978). However, in the 1980s, feminist scholarship demonstrated that resources are not shared equally within families (Pahl 1983; 1990). Women, especially if they lack an independent source of income, may be relatively deprived in terms of access to financial resources, a car, food, leisure activities and use of other valued household assets (Brannen and Wilson 1987; Deem 1986; Wimbush and Talbot 1988).

While recognizing that sharing of resources within households is unlikely to be equal, the co-resident family is nevertheless the prime arena for support of those members lacking health or an adequate personal income. In the case of ill-health or disability, practical support and care is mainly provided from within the household (Tables 3 and 4). If one household member has functional disabilities, the norm is for another household member to take on the bulk of their personal and domestic care tasks. However, caring within the household is a *resource* for the care-recipient, but may be a *constraint* for the care-giver, and in both aspects elderly women are disadvantaged relative to elderly men. Thus, although access to resources within households is gendered, there is an implicit assumption of the right to share material and caring resources. Financial and material resources are shared within households much more equally than at the levels of the community or the state.

An ideology which emphasizes reliance on the family and household assumes that everyone lives in co-resident families, or at least has relatives who are able to provide help. This assumption is increasingly challenged by recent trends. Over a quarter of households in Britain comprise only one person (Marsh and Arber 1992), and among elderly people the proportion is higher. Nearly forty per cent of elderly people live alone, with solo living two and a half times more likely for elderly women than elderly men (Table 2). For such individuals who lack material and caring resources, their only recourse is to the wider community or the state.

The community – relatives, friends and neighbours Although political rhetoric has emphasized the role of the community in supporting those in need of help, we have shown that, in practice, the bulk of 'community care' is provided within the household. Government pronouncements about community care emphasize care by friends and neighbours (Department of Health 1989), even though these sources provide only a small proportion of care to frail elderly people (Arber and Ginn 1990). However, these sources contribute to the care of elderly people living alone, providing overall, about thirteen per cent of domestic care and personal care (Tables 3 and 4).

The extent of community support for its frail members depends partly on the social characteristics of that community. The involvement of individuals in volunteer work is heavily class dependent, with twice as many middle class as working class people participating in voluntary work (Matheson 1990). More affluent areas of the country are likely to have more community resources and voluntary activity to support elderly residents than working class or deprived areas. Thus, increased reliance on the community and its volunteering capacity may lead to increasing inequalities between areas in the meeting of care needs (Leat 1986).

The state In Britain, the state is the major provider of infrastructural, health and welfare resources, and thus influences whether elderly people will be dependent on other individuals. Infra-structural resources include the level of the state retirement pension and other state benefits, the availability of adequate and appropriate housing, which maximizes independence within the individual's functional abilities, the provision of accessible and affordable public transport and the maintenance of a safe and secure outside environment. The state's provision of these resources is systematically gendered, in that it fails to meet women's greater needs. The state retirement pension, because it is flat rate, could be a powerful means of redistribution between men and women, and among classes. But its low level, below that of eligibility for means-tested benefits, means that it does little to compensate women for their sacrifice, through their caring responsibilities, of the opportunity to earn an adequate occupational pension. Although the provision of public housing, transport and a safe outside environment is equal for all elderly people, inadequacies in provision *affect* women more seriously. They are more likely to be disabled and therefore require altered accommodation, and are less likely to have access to their own car (Dale 1986) and therefore to be dependent on public transport, than men of a similar age.

The other major area of state support is provision of health care, domiciliary care and residential care. Domiciliary support services, such as home helps and meals on wheels, are vital in enabling frail elderly people to remain living in their own homes in the community. We showed earlier that domiciliary health and welfare services are not provided equally on the basis of level of disability, but are rationed according to social characteristics of the recipients, primarily the elderly person's living arrangements, but also gender ideologies about the appropriateness of providing domestic support. To the extent that future access to health care is likely to be more closely tied to having private medical insurance and to ability to pay, this will seriously disadvantage elderly women and those who have been in a poorer labour market situation during their working life.

Elderly women are more likely to reside in a communal establishment, because entering institutional care is so closely tied to widowhood or having never been married. However, although institutional care is very costly to the Exchequer, it is debatable whether it is preferred by the recipients, compared with remaining in their own home and receiving support from state domiciliary services.

Discussion

Resources enable, and lack of them constrain, an individual's activities. Our premise in this chapter is that resources are preferred at the personal level, where they are under the control of the individual, thus maximizing independence and well-being. However, the health and material resources people have at their disposal in later life is profoundly influenced by their labour market position during adult life, which is likely to have been better for men and the middle class. These structural inequalities can be substantially ameliorated by the state, but its crucial role in providing basic material support and health and social care for elderly people according to need is being eroded.

The model of a resource triangle, which is essential for the maintenance of independence and well-being, was developed in relation to elderly people, where the evidence for its gendered nature is clear. The model can also be applied to enrich our understanding of gender and class inequalities in health, in adulthood and at younger ages. Similarly, the framework which sees resources as available at four levels is equally applicable when considering the constraints and nature of dependencies created for people of all ages.

Where an individual lacks material and health resources, they are first likely to become dependent on other members of the household, who themselves may become constrained by the relationship of dependence. The provision of a state retirement pension in Britain has given elderly people a measure of independence and made them no longer reliant on their families for financial and material support (Wall 1989). Similarly, the provision of appropriate housing and accessible and affordable public transport is central to the maintenance of independence. It is a moot point whether reliance on the state for income and health or personal care allows more autonomy and independence than reliance on household members, but state support is likely to be preferred over assistance from a shifting and unreliable community. Yet the latter is the main source of practical help for elderly people who live alone, who are predominantly women.

We have seen that the state's role in providing caring services is primarily activated where an elderly person has no household members able to provide care, and few community supporters. Thus the state has a key enabling role in promoting independence of elderly people and minimizing the extent to which elderly people constrain the lives of others. Publically-funded provision of health care or domiciliary services can mitigate the effects of inequalities in health, low income or lack of informal carers, and prolong independence.

In recent years, state provision of resources has been pitted against provision by the individual, their family or the community. The 1980s and 1990s have witnessed a political movement which stresses personal responsibility, fosters individualistic self-interest, and has actively cut back the role of the state in ensuring welfare provision. The ideology of the 'New Right' centres on self-provisioning by the individual and their immediate family. Neo-liberalism and the New Right favours the purchase of social welfare services through the market (Culyer 1985), with an emphasis on privatization and voluntarism in the provision of welfare services (Leat 1986). In marketized welfare, need takes second place to purchasing power.

Thus the alternatives to state provision – either that individuals provide for their own material and caring needs or that the co-resident family or individuals in the community do so – allow the constraints of ill-health and dependency to bear hardest on those who are already disadvantaged by their previous labour market position. For those with relatively high health needs and low fixed incomes, the ideology and policies of the New Right have potentially disastrous consequences. These are more likely to affect the well-being of elderly women than elderly men, because the former are more likely to lack resources at the individual and household levels. As state provision is reduced, such structured inequalities in independence during later life will become increasingly sharp.

The most visible and distressing loss of independence – unwilling admission to an institution – is most likely to follow when all three kinds of resource are lacking; that is, if a person has insufficient income, is functionally disabled, and has no relatives who can help. Townsend (1981; 1986) argues that the social institution of residential care homes for elderly people has deprived many relatively active people of their independence. Olson goes further, linking unnecessary institutionalization in the US to poverty. Those without adequate income (predominantly women) find that their poverty and isolation often result in nursing home placement (Olson 1985:81). Elderly women's risk of institutionalization is higher than men's, an indicator of their multiple disadvantage.

Conclusion

This chapter has shown that a person's ability to live independently depends not only on their health but on two other key kinds of resources; their material resources and the informal care available to them. We do not suggest that lack of any one type of resource will necessarily threaten independence; but in combination, the likelihood of loss of home or of autonomy is multiplied. The model is equally applicable for all age groups, but has been exemplified through an analysis of structural inequalities in later life.

The resource triangle is affected by class and gender, with working class elderly people and elderly women disadvantaged in each kind of resource. Thus, structured inequalities arising from earlier biography, in terms of position in both the productive and reproductive economy, carry over into later life. Because of the constraints of their earlier domestic roles, women have to rely more heavily than men on household members and the state for financial and other material support. Their higher disability rates, combined with a greater likelihood of living alone, make them more dependent on informal care in the community and on state services. These same factors contribute to their higher rate of institutionalization, which could be seen as the ultimate loss of independence. The current attack on the welfare state is likely to magnify the effect of health inequalities, and exacerbate elderly women's disadvantage in maintaining their independence.

Acknowledgements

For access to the General Household Survey data for 1985–87 we are indebted to the ESRC Data Archive, University of Essex, and to the University of London Computer Centre. We are grateful to the Office of Population Censuses and Surveys for permission to use the GHS data. The paper is based on a research project funded by the Economic and Social Research Council (Grant No. R000231458).

References

Annandale, E. and Hunt, K. (1990), 'Masculinity, femininity and sex: an exploration of their relative contribution to explaining gender differences in health', *Sociology of Health and Illness*, **12**, (1): 24–46.

Arber, S. (1989), 'Gender and class inequalities in health: understanding the differentials', in Fox, A.J. (ed.), *Health Inequalities in European Countries*, Aldershot: Avebury.

Arber, S. (1990) 'Opening the "Black" Box: understanding inequalities in women's health', in Abbott, P. and Payne, G. (eds), *New Directions in the Sociology of Health*, Brighton: Falmer Press.

Arber, S. (1991), 'Class, paid employment and family roles: making sense of structural disadvantage, gender and health status', *Social Science and Medicine*, **32**, (4): 425–436.

Arber, S. and Ginn, J. (1990), 'The meaning of informal care: gender and the contribution of elderly people', *Ageing and Society*, **10**, (4): 429–454.

Arber, S. and Ginn, J. (1991a), *Gender and Later Life: a Sociological Analysis of Resources and Constraints*, London: Sage.

Arber, S. and Ginn, J. (1991b), 'The invisibility of age: gender and class in later life', *Sociological Review*, **39**, (2): 260–291.

Arber, S. and Ginn, J. (1992), '"In sickness and in health": care-giving, gender and the independence of elderly people', in Marsh, C. and Arber, S. (eds), *Families and Households: Divisions and Change*, London: Macmillan.

Arber, S. and Ginn, J. (1993), 'Gender and inequalities in health in later life', *Social Science and Medicine*, **36**, (1): 33–46.

Atchley, R. (1982), 'The process of retirement: comparing women and men', in Szinovacz, M. (ed.), *Women's Retirement: Policy Implications of Recent Research*, Beverly Hills: Sage.

Bearon, L.B. (1989), 'No great expectations: the underpinnings of life satisfaction of older women', *The Gerontologist*, **29**, (6): 772–784.

Braithwaite, V. (1990), *Bound to Care*, Sydney: Allen and Unwin.

Brannen, J. and Wilson, G. (eds) (1987), *Give and Take in Families*, London: Allen and Unwin.

Brody, E. (1981), '"Women in the Middle" and family help to older people', *The Gerontologist*, **21**, (5): 471–9.

Brody, E. (1985), 'Parent care as a normative family stress', *The Gerontologist*, **25**, (1): 19–29.

Central Statistical Office (1989), *Social Trends*, 19, Table 7.2, London: HMSO.

Culyer, A.J. (1985), 'On being right or wrong about the welfare state', in Bean, F., Ferris, J. and Whyness, D. (eds), *In Defence of Welfare*, London: Tavistock.

Dale, A. (1986), 'A note on differences in car usage by married men and married women', *Sociology*, **20**: 91–92.
Deem, R. (1986), *All Work and No Play: The Sociology of Women's Leisure*, Milton Keynes: Open University Press.
Department of Health and Social Security (1980), *Inequalities in Health*, The Black Report, London: DHSS.
Department of Health (1989), *Caring for people. Community care in the next decade and beyond*, Command 849, London: HMSO.
Estes, C., Swan, J. and Gerard, L. (1982), 'Dominant and competing paradigms in gerontology: towards a political economy of aging', *Ageing and Society*, **2**: 151–164.
Estes, C. (1984), 'Women and the economics of aging', *International Journal of Health Services*, **14**, (1): 55–68.
Evandrou, M. and Victor, C. (1989), 'Differentiation in later life: social class and housing tenure cleavages', in Bytheway, B., Keil, T., Allatt, P. and Bryman, A. (eds), *Becoming and Being Old: Sociological Approaches to Later Life*, London: Sage.
Finch, J. (1989), *Family Obligations and Social Change*, Cambridge: Polity Press.
Fox, A.J., Goldblatt, P. and Jones, D.R. (1983), 'Social class mortality differentials: artefact, selection or life circumstances?', *Journal of Epidemiology and Community Health*, **39**, (1): 1–18.
Fox, A.J. and Goldblatt, P. (1982), *Socio-demographic mortality differentials from the OPCS Longitudinal Study 1971–75*, Series LS, no. 1, London: HMSO.
Ginn, J. and Arber, S. (1991), 'Gender, class and income inequalities in later life', *British Journal of Sociology*, **42**, (3): 369–396.
Goldblatt, P. (1990), *Mortality and social organisation in England and Wales, 1971–1981*, Series LS, no 6, London: HMSO.
Groves, D. (1987), 'Occupational pension provision and women's poverty in old age', in Glendinning, C. and Millar, J. (eds), *Women and Poverty in Britain*, Brighton: Wheatsheaf.
Hughes, B. (1990), 'Quality of life', in Peace, S. (ed.), *Researching Social Gerontology*, London: Sage.
Land, H. (1978), 'Who cares for the family?' *Journal of Social Policy*, **7**, (3): 357–384.
Land, H. (1989), 'The construction of dependency', in Bulmer, M., Lewis, J. and Piachaud, D. (eds), *The Goals of Social Policy*, London: Unwin Hyman.
Leat, D. (1986), 'Privatisation or voluntarisation?', *Quarterly Journal of Social Affairs*, **2**, (3): 285–320.
Marsh, C. and Arber, S. (eds) (1992), *Families and Households: Divisions and Change*, London: Macmillan.
Matheson, J. (1990), *Voluntary Work*, London: HMSO.
Moser, K., Pugh, H. and Goldblatt, P. (1988), 'Inequalities in women's health: looking at mortality differentials using an alternative approach', *British Medical Journal*, **296**:1221–1224.
Mossey, J.M. and Shapiro, E. (1982), 'Self-rated health: a predictor of mortality among the elderly', *American Journal of Public Health*, **72**:800–808.
Nissel, M. and Bonnerjea, L. (1982), *Family Care of the Elderly: Who Pays?*, London: Policy Studies Institute.

Office of Population Censuses and Surveys (1987), *General Household Survey, 1985*, London: HMSO.
Olson, L. (1985), 'Older women: longevity, dependency, and public policy', in Sapiro, V. (ed.), *Women, Biology and Public Policy*, London: Sage.
Pahl, J. (1983), 'The allocation of money and the structuring of inequality within marriage', *Sociological Review*, **13**, (2): 237–262.
Pahl, J. (1990), 'Household spending, personal spending and the control of money in marriage', *Sociology*, **24**, (1): 119–138.
Palmore, E.B. and Kivett, V. (1977), 'Change in life satisfactions: a longitudinal study of persons aged 46–70', *Journal of Gerontology*, **32**, (3): 311–316.
Payne, S. (1991), *Women, Health and Poverty*, Hemel Hempstead: Harvester Wheatsheaf.
Popay, J. and Bartley, M. (1989), 'Conditions of labour and women's health', in Martin, C.J. and McQueen, D.V. (eds), *Readings for a New Public Health*, Edinburgh: Edinburgh University Press.
Shapiro, E. and Tate, R. (1988), 'Who is really at risk of institutionalisation?', *The Gerontologist*, **28**, (2): 237–245.
Singer, E., Garfinkel, R., Cohen, S.N. and Srole, L. (1976), 'Mortality and mental health: evidence from the Midtown Manhattan Restudy', *Social Science and Medicine*, **10**:517–525.
Taylor, R. (1988), 'The elderly as members of society: an examination of social differences in an elderly population', in Wells, N. and Freer, C. (eds), *The Ageing Population: Burden or Challenge?*, London: Macmillan.
Taylor, R. and Ford, G. (1983), 'Inequalities in old age: an examination of age, sex and class differences in a sample of community elderly', *Ageing and Society*, **3**, (2): 183–208.
Townsend, P. (1981), 'The structured dependency of the elderly: a creation of social policy in the twentieth century', *Ageing and Society*, **1** (1): 5–28.
Townsend, P. (1986), 'Ageism and social policy', in Phillipson, C. and Walker, A. (eds), *Ageing and Social Policy: A Critical Assessment*, Aldershot: Gower.
Ungerson, C. (1983), 'Women and caring: skills, tasks and taboos', in Gamarnikow, E., Morgan, D., Purvis, J. and Taylorson, D. (eds), *The Public and the Private*, London: Heinemann.
Victor, C. (1989), 'Health inequality in later life: age, gender or class?' in Martin, C.J. and McQueen, D.V. (eds.), *Readings for a New Public Health*, Edinburgh: Edinburgh University Press.
Victor, C. (1991), 'Change or continuity: inequalities in health in later life', *Ageing and Society*, **11**:23–39.
Victor, C. and Evandrou, M. (1987), 'Does social class matter in later life?', in di Gregorio, S. (ed.), *Social Gerontology: New Directions*, London: Croom Helm.
Wall, R. (1989), 'Leaving home and living alone: an historical perspective', *Population Studies*, **43**:369–389.
Welin, L. *et al.* (1985), 'Prospective studies of social influences on mortality', *Lancet*, **1**:915–918.
Wimbush, E. and Talbot, M. (eds) (1988), *Relative Freedoms: Women and Leisure*, Milton Keynes: Open University Press.

4 Gender differences in longevity and health in Eastern and Western Europe

Sally Macintyre

Introduction

Sex differences in health and length of life are so taken-for-granted among demographers, epidemiologists and social scientists that information on morbidity and mortality is nearly always presented separately for each sex. Anyone presenting material on rates of illness, height, mortality from heart disease, or life expectancy on both sexes combined, would immediately be asked to break down their material by gender. The fact that there are gender differences in health, and in the relationship between health and other variables, is so well known that it is standard good practice to present and analyse data separately for men and women.

Like other forms of good practice, this separate treatment of men and women can become routinized to such an extent that all curiosity about differences between men and women seems to disappear. Government publications often present sex specific statistics which are manifestly different for men and women, without providing any commentary on these differences. In the field of health inequalities, much effort is expended in developing models to explain class or regional differences; the fact that differences in morbidity or mortality between the sexes are usually greater than those between the top and bottom social strata, or the best and worst regions, is not usually commented upon. The literature on sex differences in health and life expectancy is often entirely separate from, and is not cross-referenced in, the literature on socio-economic inequalities in health.

It seems to be so taken for granted that there are sex differences (whether for social or biological reasons), that few investigators bother to study the genesis or policy implications of these differences. In this chapter, I will first describe what can be seen as the neglect of gender as a dimension in research on social inequalities in health. Secondly, I will attempt to bring gender back into the field of health inequalities, using as a focus recently available data on life expectancy among men and women in different European countries.

Gender as a neglected dimension of social differentiation in health

In the last decade there have been several major occasions on which social inequalities in health have been compared across European countries. In 1987, in Lisbon, there was a WHO Meeting of Principal Investigators on Inequities in Health. Papers from that meeting were published in a special edition of *Social Science and Medicine* (Illsley and Svensson 1990). There were contributions on inequities in health in West Germany, Finland, Britain, France, Hungary, Ireland, Israel, Italy, Malta, the Netherlands, Norway, Poland, Spain, Sweden, Switzerland, Turkey and Yugoslavia. Inequalities in many measures of morbidity and mortality were discussed by occupational social class, educational level, income, urban/rural divisions, ethnic group, region, and legitimacy (for perinatal and infant mortality rates). In most of the data, tabular material is presented separately for males and females. However, gender *per se* was not treated as a dimension of social inequalities in health or life chances.

In six of the papers, data was presented on life expectancy and changes over time in life expectancy for men and women. Gender differences in longevity (and in changes in longevity over time) were reported matter of factly and no comment or speculation offered as to the determinants of these differences. For example, the paper on West Germany gives the following commentary on a table showing life expectancy at various ages for men and women in each decade since 1950:

> In general, the German figures display the same trends as other industrialised countries both concerning the overall increase in life expectancy for males and females and the remaining and even increasing differences between the sexes. Unfortunately, in the Federal Republic life expectancy data are not registered for subgroups of the population and therefore cannot be used to identify social class differences (Kirchglasser 1990:250).

The implication of this commentary is that gender differences in longevity, and an increasing excess of female over male life expectancy, is not a matter for note or discussion. Even more striking in its apparent lack of curiosity about the data presented is the paper from Poland in which the only commentary on a life-expectancy table is:

> The trend of decrease of the average life expectancy among men, visible at the end of the 1970s, continued until the mid 1980s. Recently, there has also been a

decline in female life expectancy and this was even more intensive than among men. Both for men and women, in all age groups the average life expectancy is longer for rural residents than for inhabitants of cities (Duch and Sokolowska 1990:345).

Here, neither a trend contrary to the increase in life expectancy experienced consistently over the last century in all developed countries, nor the marked differential in the impact of this trend on the sexes, is treated as a matter to be explored, debated or investigated. Both these extracts epitomize the common treatment of gender within most of the literature on inequalities in health – the main topic of interest is whether there are social class or regional variations in mortality *among* both men and women, and is not whether, controlling for social class or region, there are differences in mortality *between* men and women.

Another special issue of *Social Science and Medicine* in 1990 focused on inequalities in health in 'non-market economies' – Bulgaria, Czechoslovakia, Hungary, Poland, and the USSR (Illsley and Wnuk-Lipinski 1990). Attention was focused on occupation, educational level and area of residence as markers of socio-economic position in countries with no 'class' systems in the traditional sense (Wnuk-Lipinski and Illsley 1990). Data on death rates and life expectancy are presented separately for males and females, but, again, sex differences are reported matter of factly and are neither commented on nor incorporated into discussions of the causes or implications of inequalities in health. For example, Eva Orosz states:

> At present the life expectancy of males at birth is identical with the level of the late 1960s and life expectancy at the age of 40 is no higher than it was in the late 1930s. International comparison of long term trends in life expectancy shows that there are not only quantitative differences between the advanced Western countries and Hungary, but that their trends have diverged from the mid 60s onward. This diverging trend is accompanied in Hungary by growing social and regional inequalities (1990:848).

A similar perspective was generally apparent in other meetings on social inequalities in health in Europe during the last decade. Between 1984 and 1986, a series of three meetings on Health Inequalities in European Countries was held in London under the auspices of the European Science Foundation and the Economic and Social Research Council. Only one paper presented in these meetings focused on gender as a dimension of inequalities (Hart 1989). Other papers focused on occupationally based measures of socio-economic position, level of education, and area of residence, with most of the emphasis being on the first of these; data were frequently presented for men and women separately but little concerted interest was shown in sex differences in the reported data. Sara Arber's interesting paper on *Gender and class inequalities in health: understanding the differentials* (Arber 1989) addressed the question of whether or not there are fewer socio-economic differentials in health for women than for men, and examined different ways of measuring socio-economic differentials among women. The intention in exploring class inequalities among women was to enhance our understanding of 'the reasons for, and pattern of, health inequalities for both men and women' (Arber 1989:276). This is a very different enterprise from one which directly explores differences between men and women, and it becomes apparent in this volume and others that terms such as 'inequalities' or 'differentials' virtually always apply to socio-economic differences in various health outcomes *among* men and women rather than to observed differences *between* men and women.

In September 1990 a meeting was held in Stockholm to discuss 'Social Equity and Health in Eastern and Western European Countries'. Background papers were prepared for Czechoslovakia, Poland, Finland, the Baltic States, Yugoslavia, Sweden, Spain, Netherlands, USSR, Bulgaria, and Romania. This meeting was extremely stimulating, coming as it did during a period in which the Eastern European countries represented were experiencing political and economic restructuring, and were revising their existing histories of the previous 40 years.

Material was presented for both Eastern and Western European countries on social inequalities in health. As with the other meetings and published collections described above, gender was nearly always incorporated into the data or analysis as a control variable, that is, in order to address the question 'does this morbidity or mortality difference by region, income, education, socio-economic strata etc occur among men and women?' In none of these papers from individual countries were differences between men and women considered directly. Yet displayed in many of these papers were marked differences, between different sorts of societies, in what had been happening to male and female life expectancy in the period since the Second World War. Consistencies within some groups of countries, and differences between these groups and others displaying a contrasting pattern, raise fascinating questions, not only about social determinants of the human lifespan but also about the distribution of roles, power, prestige and material goods to men and women in different societies. Yet the striking material presented in these papers (and described in the next section, below) was not seen as meriting particular comment or requiring further investigation. In this sense, as David Morgan has previously argued, 'Gender, as a key variable, is both ubiquitous and hidden' (Morgan 1986:31).

Sex differences in longevity in Eastern and Western Europe

Table 1 shows recent life expectancy figures for males and females, at the age of one year, in countries in Eastern and Western Europe. Eastern Europe here is a political rather than geographical concept; the countries listed are formerly communist countries from 'behind the Iron Curtain'. The data in this table predate the recent changes in political and economic structure, the dismantling of the Berlin wall and the re-unification of Germany, and the break up of the USSR.

The mean values given for Eastern and Western European countries, and for male as compared to female life expectancy, are not weighted for population size so can only be a crude indication, in particular of East/West differences. Life expectancy is higher in Western European countries than in Eastern European ones, by about 4.2 years for women and 3.8 for men. The difference between men and women is greater in Eastern European countries than in Western European countries; seven years compared to six-and-a-half years. This difference would be greater if the figures were weighted for population size, given the size of the population of the USSR and its relatively large male/female longevity difference.

Table 2 shows life expectancy for men and women in the same countries, this time giving expectation of life at the age of 45. Again, the life expectancy for males and females is greater in Western than in Eastern Europe, by 3.4 and 3.3 years. The excess of female over male life expectancy is only slightly greater in Eastern European countries – 5.6 years compared with 5.5.

Data on trends since the mid-1950s show more marked differences between different areas of Europe. Table 3 shows the increase in average life expectancy for men and women separately between 1955–60 and 1980–85. Countries in Southern Europe (Albania, Greece, Italy, Malta, Portugal, Spain and Yugoslavia) experienced the greatest increase in life expectancy for both sexes. Countries in Eastern Europe (Bulgaria, Czechoslovakia, GDR, Hungary, Poland and Romania) experienced the least increase in male life expectancy, and in these countries the gap between female and male life expectancy widened more than in other parts of Europe.

What is concealed in these 30 year trends is the consistent pattern reported from Bulgaria, Czechoslovakia, Romania, Hungary, the USSR and Poland of a deterioration in life expectancy, particularly among men in middle age, from the mid-1960s to the mid-1980s.

In Bulgaria the death rate for men in the economically active age groups grew by an average of three per cent per annum between the mid-1960s and mid-1980s. Between 1970 and 1980 the rate of male deaths per 100 female deaths rose from 114 to 120 (Minev, Dermendjéva and Mileva 1990). In Czechoslovakia, female life expectancy grew slowly but continuously between 1951 and 1985, but the male life expectancy plateaued in the early

Table 1 Life expectancy at one year of age, East and West Europe, 1980s

		Male	Female	F-M difference (years)
'Eastern' Europe				
Bulgaria	1987	68.4	74.6	6.2
Czech	1988	67.6	75.1	7.5
GDR	1988	69.4	75.5	6.1
Hungary	1988	72.0	78.6	6.6
Poland	1988	66.3	74.2	7.9
Romania	1984	67.9	73.2	5.3
USSR	1987	66.0	74.5	8.5
Yugoslavia	1987	69.4	75.1	5.7
		$\bar{x}$ = 68.8	$\bar{x}$ = 74.7	$\bar{x}$ = 6.9
'Western' Europe				
Austria	1988	71.7	78.3	6.6
Belgium	1986	71.2	77.8	6.6
Denmark	1987	71.7	77.5	5.8
Finland	1987	70.2	78.3	8.1
France	1987	72.3	80.6	8.3
GFR	1988	72.0	78.6	6.6
Greece	1986	74.1	78.7	4.6
Iceland	1988	74.0	79.4	5.4
Ireland	1987	71.3	76.8	5.5
Italy	1986	72.5	78.9	6.4
Luxemburg	1988	70.1	78.3	8.2
Netherlands	1987	73.2	79.8	6.6
Norway	1987	72.5	79.4	6.9
Portugal	1988	70.5	77.6	7.1
Spain	1985	72.9	79.3	6.4
Sweden	1987	73.7	79.8	6.1
Switzerland	1988	73.6	80.5	6.9
UK E&W	1988	72.4	78.0	5.6
UK NI	1988	70.6	76.5	5.9
UK Scotland	1988	70.2	76.3	6.1
		$\bar{x}$ = 72.0	$\bar{x}$ = 78.5	$\bar{x}$ = 6.5

Note: Statistics pre-date German reunification.

Source: WHO *Statistics Annual 1989*.

Table 2 Life expectancy at 45 years of age, East and West Europe, 1980s

		Male	Female	F-M difference (years)
'Eastern' Europe				
Bulgaria	1987	27.3	32.2	4.9
Czechoslovakia	1988	26.1	32.4	6.3
GDR	1988	27.8	32.8	5.0
Hungary	1988	25.5	32.0	6.5
Poland	1988	26.3	33.1	6.8
Romania	1984	27.4	31.5	4.1
USSR	1987	26.2	32.9	6.7
Yugoslavia	1987	28.0	32.6	4.6
		$\bar{x} = 26.8$	$\bar{x} = 32.4$	$\bar{x} = 5.6$
'Western' Europe				
Austria	1988	30.1	35.5	5.4
Belgium	1986	29.5	35.2	5.7
Denmark	1987	29.8	34.8	5.0
Finland	1987	28.8	35.4	6.6
France	1987	30.9	37.9	7.0
GFR	1988	29.9	35.7	5.8
Greece	1986	32.0	35.8	3.8
Iceland	1988	31.9	36.2	4.3
Ireland	1987	28.9	33.8	4.9
Italy	1986	30.3	35.9	5.6
Luxemburg	1988	29.0	35.4	6.4
Netherlands	1987	30.7	36.9	6.2
Norway	1987	30.5	36.4	5.9
Portugal	1988	29.8	35.1	5.3
Spain	1985	31.1	36.4	5.3
Sweden	1987	31.5	36.9	5.4
Switzerland	1988	31.9	37.7	5.8
UK E&W	1988	30.1	35.1	5.0
UK NI	1988	28.7	33.7	5.0
UK Scotland	1988	28.3	33.4	5.1
		$\bar{x} = 30.2$	$\bar{x} = 35.7$	$\bar{x} = 5.5$

Note: Statistics pre-date German reunification.

Source: WHO *Statistics Annual 1989*.

Table 3 Female–male life expectancy in 1955–60 and 1980–85, and increases in life expectancy over this period, in different parts of Europe

Part of Europe	Years		*Male increase (years)*	*Female increase (years)*
	F-M, 1955–60	*F-M, 1980–85*		
Eastern	4.6	7.0	3.0	5.4
Northern	5.2	6.0	3.2	4.0
Western	5.4	7.3	3.8	5.7
Southern	4.2	6.1	6.7	8.6

Source: Zvidrins, P. and Krumins, P. 1990, Appendix 1.

1960s and then declined. The male life expectancy experienced in 1964 was only attained again in 1987 (Janeckova and Hnilicova 1990). Janeckova and Hnilicova compare male life expectancy in 1974–75 and 1984–87 in various countries and show that Bulgarian, Romanian, Polish and Hungarian men all experienced decreasing life expectancy in this period. A similar comparison for women shows that life expectancy increased less in these same countries (plus the USSR) than in other countries (Janeckova and Hnilicova 1990).

Eva Orosz has pointed out that while in Western Europe health and life expectancy has in general improved since the Second World War, though with continuing disparities between socio-economic strata, in Hungary mortality rates deteriorated from the mid-1960s onwards, particularly for males. In the mid-1960s the growth in life expectancy in males stopped; it stagnated and slightly declined until the mid-1970s, then drastically declined. At the end of the 1980s, the life expectancy of males at birth was identical with the level of the late 1950s, while their life expectancy at 40 was no higher than it was in the 1930s. Table 4 shows how age-standardized mortality rates of men and women have risen since 1960, the male rates rising faster than the female rates (by 4.3 per 1000 compared to 2.8 per 1000) (Orosz 1990).

Crude and age-standardized mortality rates also rose among men in the USSR from the mid-1960s. The age-standardized male mortality rate increased from 12.6 in 1970 to 14.1 in 1980. Table 5 shows life expectancy in the USSR for males and females from 1960–61 to 1986–87. It was only in the late 1980s that men's life expectancy was back up to its 1960 level. Women's life expectancy fluctuated around 73 years, increasing in the late 1980s to nearer 74 years. In the 1970s the female/male gap in life expect-

Table 4 Age-standardized mortality rates (per 1,000) by sex in Hungary, since 1930

Year	Males	Females
1930–31	16.9	15.2
1948–49	12.5	10.6
1959–60	10.9	9.7
1969–70	12.3	10.7
1979–80	14.3	12.1
1984–85	15.2	12.5

Source: Orosz 1990.

Table 5 Life expectancy at birth for males and females, 1960–87, USSR

Year	Males	Females
1960–61	65.3	72.7
1970–71	64.5	73.5
1980–81	62.3	72.5
1982–83	62.8	73.0
1984–85	62.9	72.7
1986–87	65.0	73.8

Source: Mezentseva and Rimachevskaya 1990.

ancy at birth was ten years, one of the highest in the world. By 1987 it was 8.8 years (Mezentseva and Rimachevskaya 1990).

In Poland mortality rates, which had been dropping for 20 years, started rising again in the mid-1970s. A decrease in men's life expectancy started in the mid-1970s and continued until the mid-1980s. During the 1980s women's life expectancy started to decline, at a rate even faster than men's. Between 1980 and 1985, the difference between men and women in mortality rates narrowed because of this rise in women's mortality (Duch and Sokolowska 1990).

Discussion

There is thus consistent evidence that while life expectancy was consistently increasing in Western European countries over the four decades from 1950 to 1990, life expectancy in Eastern European countries was stagnating or declining, especially among males. Such a consistent and marked pattern in changes in the length of human life is very striking. The fact that it has not received more attention may be due to a number of factors, including the fact that health statistics in many Eastern European countries have tended to focus on input measures (number of doctors or hospital beds) rather than output measures (morbidity or mortality).

One reason for this lack of interest in sex differences in health may be the assumption that the differences are fixed, possibly because of biological factors, and therefore not a proper topic for sociological enquiry. Yet examination of sex differences in life expectancy, (which is, after all, one of the 'hardest' health measures of all, and the one least subject to artefactual biases), reveals sufficient historical and cross-cultural variation to indicate that it is subject to social, political, economic or cultural influences. According to Hart (1989; 1990), most evidence suggests that from the early palaeolithic period to the beginnings of the industrial revolution men had a longer life span (at around 40 years) than women (at around 35 years). Excess female mortality was not confined to the childbearing years but seems to have been present from the early teens. With industrialization, women's life expectancy first equalled, then outstripped, men's, so that women in most industrialized countries can now expect to live six years longer on average than men. Males have higher rates of foetal death, stillbirth and neonatal deaths, and it is likely that this male excess mortality in the first stages of life has always been common. It is thus not the explanation for greater female than male life expectancy at birth, and indeed excess male mortality rates are now found at all points of the life span in industrialized societies (Hart 1989).

In some societies, men still live longer on average than women; in the 1970s and 1980s men's life expectancy was greater than, or very close to, women's in a number of countries, mainly in the Indian sub-continent (India, Pakistan, Bangladesh, Nepal, Bhutan, Afghanistan, Iran, Tunisia and the Maldives (WHO 1989)). This female excess of deaths is not confined to the periods of early infancy and/or childbearing, so does not seem solely attributable either to early neglect of females or to particularly adverse circumstances for reproduction.

Presentation of such exceptions to the currently more common pattern of longer female life expectancy often provokes the response that these figures are somehow distortions (because of poverty, or cultural attitudes to women) of the 'natural' pattern. This begs the question of what a 'natural' pattern of male/female differences in life expectancy is, and how one could ascertain this. Is the pattern that Hart (1990) argues has persisted for 99 per cent human evolution – males and females living a relatively short time, and males living longer than women – the 'natural' one, with modern patterns a distortion because of industrialization and 'artificial' sex role obligations? Or are we moving towards a more 'natural' pattern as we progressively get rid of 'artificial' constraints such as scarcity and wars?

The issue of the naturalness of male/female differences in longevity may itself seem artificial, but its importance lies in the way in which implicit concepts of naturalness underpin our reaction to, and interpretation of, male/female mortality rates, and our frequent failure to consider the origins or implications for policy of such differences. Changes in longevity, and in the balance between male and female longevity, in Eastern Europe and Western Europe over the last 40 years, raise questions about the responsiveness of the human life span to social and economic circumstances; about the differential vulnerability of men and women to socio-economic circumstances; and about the allocation of roles, power, prestige and material goods to men and women in different societies.

Although investigators in the field of inequalities in health rarely directly address gender differences, there is of course a specific literature on gender difference in health and illness (Nathanson 1984; Verbrugge 1985; Waldron 1976). What is a matter for some regret is that the two bodies of literature, inequalities and sex differences in health, are so separate. Studies of one dimension of social differentiation in health – for example, social class – might have much to learn from studies of other dimensions such as gender.

What does the literature on sex differences in health tell us? Although in industrialized societies women live longer than men, they have higher rates of morbidity. In the UK and USA it has been consistently found that women have higher rates of physical illness, disability days, use of prescribed and non-prescribed medication, and contact with physicians, even when one removes conditions or health behaviour directly related to childbirth. (Detailed reviews are provided by Verbrugge 1985 and 1989, and Waldron 1976 and 1982.) Data from America show a sex difference in the incidence of acute conditions of around 20–30 per cent overall, women having excess morbidity for all major groups of conditions. Most non-fatal chronic disease is also more common among women. Women restrict their activities for health reasons about 25 per cent more days, and spend on average 40 per cent more days in bed, per year than men. Sex differences in use of health services are greatest in the childbearing years (in the age range 17–44 women have about twice as many physician visits per year as men). When reproductive and other specifically sex-linked conditions are excluded, there is still an excess of about 30 per cent for outpatient care, but women's and men's hospitalization rates become very similar. Women obtain significantly more prescription, especially psychotropic, drugs than men, and also report using more over-the-counter medications (Verbrugge 1985).

Men show health disadvantages in fewer, but perhaps more life-threatening, conditions. Between the ages of 17 and 44 men have 50 per cent more accidents than women. They are more likely to have impairments (some resulting from accidents) than women. Long term disability due to chronic health problems, which interferes with major life activities such as paid work or parenting roles, is more common among men, especially at older ages. Men have higher prevalence rates for potentially fatal conditions such as coronary heart disease, atherosclerosis, and emphysema (Verbrugge 1985).

In sum, in the USA and in Western European countries such as the UK for which similar data are available, women have more frequent illness and disability, and use more health care resources than men, while men suffer more from life-threatening diseases which may cause more permanent disability and earlier death. The initially paradoxical finding that men die earlier than women, but suffer less illness and disability, seems less paradoxical when the *types* of illness and disabilities commonly reported by both sexes are taken into account.

There are a number of possible explanations for the differences between men and women in reported rates of illness, disability, and use of services. The most commonly cited are:

i) biological risks, i.e. those inherent in physiological characteristics of the sexes;
ii) acquired risks, i.e. risks of illness and injury arising from different behaviour patterns (such as rates of driving, smoking, recreational or work-based exercise, or alcohol consumption) or from differential exposure to physical or psychological hazards;
iii) health reporting behaviour, i.e. differential tendencies to perceive symptoms of illness and distress, and to act upon these or to report them to health workers or interviewers;
iv) health care, i.e. different access to, use of, or treatment by the health care system.

These different types of explanation have been extensively reviewed and examined by Verbrugge (1985). In her very interesting recent work she shows that if one controls for health reporting behaviour and for acquired risks (including role position and socio-economic status), then the usual pattern of higher female rates of morbidity reverses; that is, men then show higher rates of (less serious) illness and disability. Although biological risks were not studied directly, she suggests that women's apparent excess in morbidity is, in large part, determined by their social roles and that, given similar social circumstances, men might display more vulnerability to physical or psychological threats (Verbrugge 1988, 1989).

Most of the published work on sex differences in illness, disability and use of health services comes from outside Eastern Europe. Many of the explanations for observed differences are based on the expectation of sex-segregated roles, in particular that women are more likely to be home-makers and that men are more likely to be in paid employment (hence hypotheses about 'fixed' and 'nurturant' roles, e.g. Gove 1984). It would be very interesting to know whether similar gender differences have been apparent over the last three decades in Eastern European countries, in which women have been more likely to have been in paid employment than they have in Western European countries (and to have been employed in occupations such as medicine, which in Western European countries are male dominated). Unfortunately such morbidity data by gender are not readily available.

This chapter has attempted to raise questions about gender differences in mortality and morbidity, and about their relationship to social structure and social conditions, rather than to answer them. The data summarized have a number of implications both for our understanding of the social determinants of health and longevity and for our ideas about the equitable distribution of health care and other resources.

Considering firstly the social determinants of health and longevity, five main questions arise. Firstly, how are we to explain the increasing male/female gap in longevity in industrialized countries? Is it increasing because men are exposed to more potentially lethal risks than women, or because women are physiologically more robust and survive better when exposed to similar risks to men? One hypothesis is that:

> increasing equality between the sexes in various areas of life, particularly in work, and the concomitant convergence of life styles, result in a narrowing of the sex mortality differential (Koskinen *et al.* 1989:1–2).

This hypothesis has recently been tested on Finnish data and found not to be supported (Javanainen 1989; Koskinen *et al.* 1989). An alternative hypothesis is that males are intrinsically more vulnerable than females (as evidenced by higher foetal death, stillbirth and neonatal death rates), and that if there were to be increasing equality between the sexes in the distribution between them of roles, risks, power, prestige and material resources, males would experience higher morbidity and mortality than women (Verbrugge 1985; Hart 1990). More research needs to be conducted on these competing hypotheses.

Secondly, why did men's mortality stagnate or increase from the mid-1960s in Eastern European countries but women's mortality continued to decline steadily? What are the social and physical circumstances in which improving longevity for women co-existed with deteriorating longevity for men? One hypothesis might relate to the second of the two hypotheses mentioned in the previous paragraph; namely that if males are in some way more vulnerable than females, adverse social and material conditions of living, which might have existed in these countries from the mid-1960s, might be expected to have a greater impact on male than on female mortality.

Thirdly, over the last few decades were the gender differences in illness, disability and use of health services in Eastern European countries similar to those in Western European countries? Did the relatively greater participation of women in the labour force lessen or increase differences between the sexes? What effect did the 'double burden' – of paid work and domestic responsibilities – have on women's health, especially in societies with few labour saving devices?

Fourthly, and relatedly, what will happen to men's and women's mortality and morbidity rates with the political and economic changes now taking place in these formerly non-market economies? A common expectation is that with the move to a market economy, many women will retreat, or be extruded, from the labour market; and also that occupations such as medicine will rise in status and pay and become more masculinized. If these trends do happen, what will be the impact on the sex differences in health and length of life?

Finally, are the processes which lead to sex differentials in health and longevity the same as, or different from, those which lead to differentials by socio-economic factors? Because sex differences are so often simultaneously taken-for-granted and ignored in the inequalities in health field, such a question is rarely asked but, as I have previously argued (Macintyre 1986), it is an important one to address, because models of social determinants of health can be refined or expanded by looking at a number of types of inequalities such as by sex, socio-economic status, region of the country and so on.

Considering the implications for health and social policy, two main questions can be asked: firstly, what weight should health policies give to morbidity as compared with mortality; and what weight should it give to prevention as compared with care or cure? These questions are not gender-neutral. If one focuses on morbidity and looks at male/female differences, one might decide that resources should be devoted to making women as healthy as men; if one focuses on mortality, one might decide to devote resources to helping men live as long as women. A focus on prevention would put resources into heart disease as a problem of premature male mortality; a focus on care might allocate more resources to heart disease and strokes among elderly women.

Secondly, what do we mean by equity in health care? Gavin Mooney has identified seven possible definitions of equity: equality of expenditure per capita; equality of inputs per capita; equality of input for equal need; equality of access for equal need; equality of utilization for equal need;

equality of marginal met need; and equality of health. He examines the issues surrounding these definitions and points out that the last definition, that of equality of health, requires much greater positive discrimination in health care provision than any of the definitions based on input, and would involve an extremely unequal distribution of health care resources (Mooney 1983). These sorts of definitions of equity have mainly been considered in relation to the allocation of resources between regions, but form a useful framework for thinking about what we might mean by equity in relation to socio-economic strata or to the sexes. There is, too, the further issue of whether equity, whether between socio-economic strata, regions, or sexes, should be a goal of health care provision or social policy. While lip service is given to equity or equality in health as a goal by many countries, particularly in relation to targets for Health For All by the Year 2000, it is unclear to what extent the concept of health equalities is now discredited in formerly non-market economies, as suggested by Orosz (1990).

In conclusion, I suggest that sex differentials in morbidity and mortality should be incorporated into research and thinking about social inequalities in health. While some sex differences may have underlying biological causes, it is impossible to imagine the expression of these causes as being separable from the social and physical environment. Data on longevity provide striking evidence of the variability of male and female life chances according to social conditions. Rather than treating sex differences as 'given', or 'fixed', we should confront these differences and explore their implications for our understanding of the determinants of health; our understanding of the distribution of power, prestige, roles, risks and material resources within societies; and for the planning of health and social policy.

Acknowledgements

I am grateful to Gill Green and Anne Sooman in gathering some of the data presented in earlier versions of this paper, to participants in the East–West workshop for their papers and for their comments on an earlier draft, and to Jean Leiper for typing the manuscript.

References

Arber, S. (1989), 'Gender and class inequalities in health: understanding the differentials', in Fox, J. (ed.), *Health Inequalities in European Countries*, Aldershot: Avebury.

Duch, D. and Sokolowska, M. (1990), 'Health inequalities in Poland', *Social Science and Medicine*, **31**:343–350.

Gove, W.R. (1984), 'Gender differences in mental and physical illness: the effects of fixed roles and nurturant roles', *Social Science and Medicine*, **19**:77–91.
Hart, N. (1989), 'Sex, gender and survival: inequalities of life chances between European men and women', in Fox, J. (ed.), *Health Inequalities in European Countries*, Aldershot: Avebury.
Hart, N. (1990), 'Female vitality and the history of human health', paper presented to Third International Conference of the European Society for Medical Sociology, Marburg.
Illsley, R. and Svensson, P.-G. (eds) (1990), 'Health inequities in Europe' – *special issue*, *Social Science and Medicine*, **31**:223–420.
Illsley, R. and Wnuk-Lipinski, E. (eds) (1990), 'Non-market economies in health', *Social Science and Medicine*, **31**:831–889.
Janeckova, H. and Hnilicova, H. (1990), 'The health status of the Czechoslovak population: its social and ecological determinants', paper prepared for the East–West Workshop on Social Equity and Health in Europe, Stockholm, September.
Javanainen, M. (1989), *Convergence of life styles and sex ratio in suicide mortality in Finland*, Working Paper No. 46, Department of Sociology, University of Helsinki.
Kirchgassler, K-U. (1990), 'Health and social inequities in the Federal Republic of Germany', *Social Science and Medicine*, **31**:249–526.
Koskinen, S., Valkonen, T., Martikainen, P. and Martolin, T. (1989), *Convergence of life styles and trends in sex mortality ratio among the middle aged in Finland*, Working Paper No. 44, Department of Sociology, University of Helsinki.
Macintyre, S. (1986), 'The patterning of health by social position in contemporary Britain: directions for sociological research', *Social Science and Medicine*, **23**:393–415.
Mezentseva, E. and Rimachevskaya, N. (1990), 'The Soviet country profile: health of the USSR population in the 70s and 80s', *Social Science and Medicine*, **31**:867–877.
Minev, D., Dermendjeva, B. and Mileva, N. (1990), 'The Bulgarian country profile: the dynamics of some inequalities in health', *Social Science and Medicine*, **31**:837–846.
Mooney, G. (1983), 'Equity in health care: confronting the confusion', *Effective Health Care*, **1**:178–184.
Morgan, D. (1986), 'Gender', in Burgess, R. (ed.), *Key Variables in Social Investigation*, London: Routledge and Kegan Paul.
Nathanson, C. (1984), 'Sex differences in mortality', *Annual Review of Sociology*, **10** (eds Turner, R.H. and Short, J.F.):191–213.
Orosz, E. (1990), 'The Hungarian country profile: inequalities in health and health care in Hungary', *Social Science and Medicine*, **31**:847–857.
Verbrugge, L.M. (1985), 'Gender and health: an update on hypotheses and evidence', *Journal of Health and Social Behaviour*, **26**:156–182.
Verbrugge, L.M. (1988), 'Unveiling higher morbidity for men', in Riley, M.W. with Huber, B.J. and Hess, B.B. (eds), *Social Structures and Human Lives*, London: Sage Publications.
Verbrugge, L.M. (1989), 'The twain meet: empirical explanations of sex differences in health and mortality', *Journal of Health and Social Behaviour*, **30**:282–304.

Waldron, I. (1976), 'Why do women live longer than men?' *Social Science and Medicine*, **10**:349–62.
Waldron, I. (1982), 'An analysis of causes of sex differences in mortality and morbidity', in Gove, W.R. and Carpenter, G.R. (eds), *The Fundamental Connection between Nature and Nurture*, Lexington: Lexington Books.
Wnuk-Lipinski, E. and Illsley, R. (1990), 'Introduction', *Social Science and Medicine*, **31**:833–836.
World Health Organisation (1989), *Statistics Annual 1989*, Geneva: World Health Organisation.
Zvidrins, P. and Krumins, J. (1990), 'Morbidity and mortality in Estonia, Latvia and Lithuania in the 80s', paper prepared for East–West Workshop on Social Equity and Health, Stockholm, September.

5 Feminism and the health consequences of women's work in late nineteenth and early twentieth century Britain

Barbara Harrison

Introduction

This chapter examines the women's movement or feminist activism during the period of 'first wave feminism' that spans the 1880s through to the end of the first decade of the twentieth century. It has been argued that there are considerable problems with traditional analyses of these early feminists, not only because attention is given to specific aspects of organization, such as that around trade unionism or suffrage but also in the characterization of it as a whole (Levine 1988; Walby 1990). These same accounts have sought to re-evaluate the nature of Victorian feminism in terms of the issues with which it was concerned, the origins of its activists, particularly in terms of class, and its success as a political movement. Walby (1990) has criticized the characterization of 'first wave feminism' as being middle class, pursuing a narrow range of interests, namely suffrage, within a liberal political philosophy of rights. On the contrary, she argues, this is an injustice to a feminism which was concerned with a wide range of demands, and the interests of all women from a variety of political positions. It was in effect 'a large multi-faceted, long lived and highly effective political phenomena' (Walby 1990:97). If we accept the validity of this portrayal of previous scholarship, it opens for further investigation and discussion aspects of feminist activism without necessarily being curtailed by existing frames of reference, although some of these will remain relevant. Feminism is beginning to deal with the contradictions and divisions which cut across the notion of gender as a class and 'sisterhood' as an all-encompassing political movement (Ramazanoglu 1989). In examining industrial ill health within an analysis of 'first wave feminism', we can begin to appreciate the shifting alliances of 'sisterhood' that cut across dimensions such as class.

My specific aim is to explore the place of one particular issue – the health consequences of women's working conditions – within feminism at this time: to analyse the significance of health as an issue within feminism and feminist responses to it. Having for some time researched women's occupational ill health in this period, it seemed necessary to pursue this particular dimension for a number of reasons. First, although there has been a considerable amount written about 'protective' legislation, both as a form of state intervention in working women's lives and also as a focus for feminist activity, the interest has tended to focus on what it tells us about divisions within feminism (Banks 1981; Feurer 1988). In such analyses while working conditions generally feature as a context for a discussion of views on legislation as a remedy, the political struggles are not viewed as being essentially about health. Thus 'protective' legislation itself has been given a particular significance and meaning. It seemed necessary to ask different questions: To what extent did feminist analysis and political practice around women's work at this time take the health consequences of work to be a serious issue? How was it viewed and defined and what were the consequences?

Second, it did seem evident from my research thus far that women's health was indeed affected, most often adversely, by aspects of their paid employment as well as the interrelationship of paid and unpaid work. In the public domain there was a discourse around the health consequences for women and their families of industrial work, which by the end of the century had become part of a changing social and political climate in which state intervention was perceived as a moral responsibility for the failure of the industrial system to fulfil its commitment to human capital. Reproductive health, motherhood and child health were central concerns in official circles and outside. Women's work was perceived to threaten the nation's health. If these issues were prominent in the public domain, then one might expect there to have been a feminist response to them.

Finally, occupational ill health itself has been a marginal issue, at least in scholarship, since neither an interest in the health of women or their working lives has seemed to adequately encompass it. There was also the possibility that for feminist practice it was also a marginal issue and that scholarship had simply reflected this. It was an assumption that required examination.

Many writers have alluded to the difficult task of rendering aspects of women's history visible (Rowbotham 1977; Scott 1988). This work is no exception. The primary and secondary sources used leave many women's voices silent. It is difficult to gain any sense of how working class women, those by and large engaged in the employments with which I have been concerned, felt or thought about their work, health and other aspects of their lives, except through other peoples representations of them.[1] Despite this it is important to attempt to render a corrigible, interpretative account of experience or otherwise we compound the invisibility. Although it is not possible to debate these here, I am aware that this raises epistemological issues such as those discussed by feminist scholars around the category 'woman' (Harding 1987; Riley 1988; Stanley 1990) and the extent to which historical discourse itself has become imbued with categories derived from its own objects of study, particularly forms of political struggle (Scott 1987).

Late nineteenth century feminism and 'protective' legislation

Before moving on to an examination of health in the context of 'protective' legislation and feminist politics, it is necessary to outline the main groups involved, the essence of the positions they took toward 'protective' legislation and the meaning of 'protective' legislation. This term has been used to describe the underlying rationale of state intervention in the industrial system, through legislation principally aimed at factories and mines. Early in the nineteenth century, the stated intention was to protect children, but by the 1840s women were to be included in such legislation on the grounds that they, like children, were in need of special protection because of their perceived physical and political vulnerability. From 1842, when women were excluded from underground mine work, factory legislation continued to enact regulations which applied only to children, young persons and women. Underlying the principle of the need to protect women as a special class was a concern not only with limiting the effects of work on them, but also, more importantly, on their domestic roles and their ability to care for the health of their husbands and children. By the end of the nineteenth century, the idea of 'protection' in these terms resulted in increasing public agitation and official investigation in order to establish the problems of working conditions, and to possibly remove women, especially married women, from considerable areas of the labour market. It was, therefore, not necessarily the intention of factory legislation to protect the health of workers: its purpose was to protect the health of the nation from the dangers of women at work (Harrison and Mockett 1990).

There are limitations in dividing the discussion of late nineteenth century feminism into two divergent 'camps' – equal rights feminists and social feminists – according to whether they opposed or supported 'protective' legislation. Constant changes in organization took place, and there were shifts within and across these two strands over time. These are briefly summarized here.

Prior to the late 1880s, while there were different forms of political philosophy and organizations which represented these, there was a united opposition to the idea of state interference with women's labour. Equal rights feminists had been active in campaigns before the period examined here, and their organizational base had been formed in the 1860s and 1870s. These organizations, such as the Society for the Employment of Women (SPEW) and the Vigilance Association for the Defence of Personal Rights (VA) combined philanthropic concerns with widening employment opportunities for women and opposition to legal restrictions. They also had the periodical the *English Woman's Journal*, later to become the *English Woman's Review* (EWR) to publicize their causes (Murray and Clarke 1985). Their overall political philosophy was concerned in general with equal rights, personal freedom and 'laissez faire' policies in social and economic matters. State intervention would thus make women more dependent and defenceless and the Factory Acts, like other laws, were degrading to women, exacerbating economic and political powerlessness. In their view, gender was a class, and their opposition to all forms of patriarchal control was evident. One of their main arguments against a male legislature restricting women's work was that it reflected male fears of competition. Jessie Boucherett commenting on the Report of the House of Lords Select Committee on Homework in 1890, noted:

> The Committee acknowledges men's complaints are not genuine, and then proceeds to endorse them, and recommends that these poor women should be forbidden.... Legislation for the assumed object of preventing women from over-working themselves, and for the real object of competing with men is unfair (*English Woman's Review*, (EWR), 16 June, 1890:248).

Until the 1890s, social feminism encompassed a variety of trade union, labour and socialist political organizations and were also opposed to state intervention.[2] Social feminists agreed with the view that fear of competition was a motive in men's attempts to restrict women's employment. On numerous occasions, particularly within the Trades Union Congress (TUC), they found themselves having to defend a woman's right to work against male unionist calls for the state to exclude them. In 1887, for example, Clementina Black in opposing a motion calling for 'the prevention of the employment of females in the chain and nail making trades', argued:

> That women did suffer the physical evils was no doubt true. But there was not one injury which Mr Juggins had instanced that could not be capped by a worse story of the women employed in trades no one dreamed of forbidding, such as needlework and matchbox making. Why not? There was no need to ask. Men did not work at these trades and suffered nothing from the competition of women (*Women's Union Journal*, 15 Oct., 1887:141 xii).

The primary focus for social feminism until the 1890s had been to encourage the formation of women's unions. Equal rights feminists had also supported goals of unionization and the need for separate women's organizations. They were to join with organizations such as the Women's Provident and Protective League (WPPL) in campaigns against state interference, notably that around women's pitbrow work in the 1880s. Both groups also actively campaigned for the appointment of women to the Factory Department. It is important to note that most social feminists were campaigning for working women with direct knowledge and experience of working conditions to become inspectors (Jones 1988), although it was eventually middle class women who were appointed. Finally, neither disputed the awful nature of women's working conditions.

This was to change from the late 1880s. The sometimes bitter division that was evident between the two groups from here on was a consequence of changes within social feminism and its organizations.[3] The major transformation around social feminist thinking and strategy was the abandonment of its faith in women's unionism for the time being, and its opposition to 'protective' legislation. A new practical politics was considered necessary to remedy the continuing exploitation and conditions of the working woman. New organizations evolved (in particular the Women's Industrial Council (WIC), the Women's Labour League (WLL), the Women's Cooperative Guild, and later the Fabian Women's Group (FWG)) which focused on all questions relating to women's employment and industrial conditions, and they became involved in investigation as well as political campaigning (Mappen 1985, 1986).

This change in social feminism can be attributed to two main factors. Firstly, their increasing acquaintance with actual working conditions. They were, in Clementina Black's words, 'shocked and horrified' by what they saw. Secondly, a growth in union consciousness, influenced by 'new unionism' and a closer relationship of women's organizations to the TUC. An ascendancy of socialist ideas within this context gave rise to a new political perspective on working conditions. Although social feminists now favoured state intervention as a means of remedy, it should not be assumed that this was wholehearted. Many still questioned the motives of men who supported it, and there were some who argued against the gender-specific nature of the legislation. As Enid Stacey put it:

> ...a great injustice will be done to women if state interference deals with them intimately and leaves men pretty much alone. Socialists urge that the state has power to regulate individuals *qua* individuals but not *qua* women (cited in Levine 1987:120; emphasis in the original).

This position on legislation was consistent with an increasing emphasis on class as well as gender goals. Although women workers were seen to have special needs and to occupy a particular position in the labour market, they favoured strategies which would benefit all workers. In the event, many social feminists found themselves supporting gender-specific legislation rather than foregoing the possibility of reform at all.

Within equal rights feminism, there were few visible shifts in analysis, organization or political strategy. In every case, including women's working conditions, the law was viewed consistently as an attempt to limit women's opportunities and to interfere with their personal liberty. They remained hostile to the motives of male unionists and the state alike, and viewed the 'new' politics of social feminism as collusion with them. Their unshakeable belief in 'freedom' brought considerable criticism, and by the time the split came with social feminism, they were being accused of colluding with employers in their exploitation of women, and of exposing women to unnecessary dangers in the workplace. There was also the suspicion that their main interest was in freedom for middle class women, not their hard-pressed working class 'sisters'. Beatrice Webb (1902), in one such attack, accused middle class women of 'blacklegging'. However, we also need to remember that equal rights feminists saw work opportunities as paramount, and consistently supported those rights for *all* women. They were correct in their perception that a state strategy aimed at restricting women's employment was one which would perpetuate discrimination within the labour market and outside.

These divisions within nineteenth century feminism have been frequently cast as divisions of class, not least by activists themselves at the time. There were some differences in the class interests that assumed priority at particular times, but both were concerned with working class women. The leadership in both cases, and to a considerable extent their membership, was middle class. There were more working women involved with social feminism, especially within the Women's Trade Union League (WTUL); and it is probably not unfair to characterize equal rights feminism as being more involved with employment goals for middle class women than social feminists. There were undoubtedly ways in which class was a salient feature of feminist activism, but it would be a mistake to consider allegiances and political analysis and practice solely in these terms. Gender and class both united and pulled feminists in different directions.

Working conditions and health: documenting the toll

It is impossible to do justice to the range of working conditions and their consequences to health, that were shown to exist in this period, and it is to women factory inspectors and feminist activism that we owe much of this information. The commitment to investigation within social feminism gave them and the public domain considerable data on the scale of grievances about conditions. The Women's Cooperative Guild and the Women's Industrial Council undertook numerous investigations into the trades, although their reports' contents demonstrate that economic issues, rather than health considerations, tended to be of paramount concern. Investigation is less evident within equal rights feminism, but their use of periodical outlets, such as the various suffrage journals and the aforementioned *English Woman's Review*, did provide opportunities to do so.

Social feminist organizations thus became an outlet for working women to voice their grievances. The WTUL, for example, not only collected such grievances for informational or propaganda purposes, but acted as a channel for such complaints to reach the inspectorate. These complaints helped to identify products, processes and environmental aspects, as well as the problems of long hours and illegal overtime as causing ill health in women.

Perhaps the most vivid accounts of working conditions are to be found in the reports of the women factory inspectors. Prior to their appointment, a precedent was set in the specialist investigation of women's working conditions and their effects on their 'health, morality and the home' by the appointment of Assistant Lady Commissioners to the Royal Commission on Labour in 1893. The four commissioners investigated workplaces all over the country, from white lead works, to tailoring, public houses and hotels, textile mills to tailoring shops, and so on. In addition to the work of investigating complaints and routine inspection, women inspectors conducted numerous special investigations. Inspectors reports not only give a sense of the nature of their own work, they also indicate the range of workplaces covered, the kinds of problems they were prepared to countenance, and their own particular analysis of what could contribute to women's ill health. The work of the inspectors also represented a departure from 'officially' recognized problems, as evidenced in legislation. Thus, although they did considerable work on the 'dangerous trades', their own priorities were often for improvements in sanitary conditions, ventilation, extreme cold and heat, the lifting of heavy weights, and the continuing problems of hours of work. They also drew attention to the exploitation of women in terms of violence and sexual harassment (Lambertz 1985), and through systems of fines and deductions, and payment in kind.

The decision of the state to respond to demands for further intervention also led to an unprecedented level of official investigation in the form of Committees of Inquiry and Royal Commissions. The evidence presented and the reports' findings also provide rich sources of information. Finally, by the 1890s, a number of medical practitioners began to devote themselves to the identification of industrial disease and in their own writing gave some attention to women's occupations (Arlidge 1892; Oliver 1902). Oliver's work on the dangerous trades is interesting in two respects: he used women inspectors to write up some chapters on particular women's trades, presumably in recognition of specialist expertise, and he devoted a whole chapter to domestic servants. This reminds us of the limitations of information generated in a context of state intervention, and although feminists did consider working conditions more widely than those found in the factory, workshop or home, this was inevitably less politically pressing than those where interference was proposed or thought desirable. The largest sector of employed women workers, domestic servants, thus remained outside of public, feminist and official consciousness alike, even though their conditions were frequently no less damaging to health.

Women inspectors, feminism and health

It is not usual to include within the feminist movement at this time, the women factory inspectors, but, while there might be a case for this, it does seem important to examine their relation to it.[4] This is particularly so in relation to health and working conditions. We have demonstrated above that both equal rights and social feminists supported the campaigns for women to be appointed as factory inspectors. It is possible that this was for different political reasons, although they were certainly united on the value of women and their special skills in the inspection and investigation of women's work. There are a number of reasons to suppose that the links between the inspectors and feminists extended beyond the value of their official role to feminist practical politics. There were friendship networks between members of the WTUL and the early women inspectors.[5] A number of inspectors also had links with social feminist organizations prior to or while they worked in the inspectorate, and we know that inspectors often appeared on their public platforms as contributors. They saw such involvement as part of their own strategy of increasing working women's knowledge about conditions, and their rights under factory legislation. Social feminists also acted as a channel for complaints to be investigated by the inspectorate, and up to one-third of all complaints came from these sources. (For a more detailed examination of the work of the female inspectorate see McFeely 1988; Jones 1988 and their own autobiographical accounts, Anderson 1922; Squire 1927; Martindale 1944.)

The inspectorate also gave impetus to feminist demands for increased employment opportunities for middle class women in professional and official occupations. It has been suggested (Jones 1988) that their success here may have been greater than in ameliorating conditions for working class women. Rose Squire (1927) recollected that not only was it expected that daughters of professional men should not take up careers, but inspection was viewed as 'not quite nice', an 'unladylike' occupation, and such views were evident in the early debates about the desirability of appointing women. Inspectors encountered sexism in numerous ways throughout their work and shared other feminists' frustrations over the degree of control men exercised over the decisions which affected the lives of women. In this, their sympathy with the suffrage cause was evident. Rose Squire cites the example of discussions at the Home Office on the proposed 1895 Factory and Workshop Bill:

> It seemed to me irksome that men, ignorant for the most part of the words they uttered took part in the discussion, while I, who knew so much, had to impart a few hasty sentences (Squire 1927:27).

As with other feminist activists, the women's inspectorate strongly resisted forms of regulation which were exclusionary or prohibitory in nature, although they argued this might be right on public grounds. In evidence to the 1908/9 committee on the potteries, Adelaide Anderson replied to the proposed restriction on pregnant women and nursing mothers that:

> Enquiries I have made or caused to be made have shown that in 9 cases out of 10, they go back (to work) because of some strong domestic or economic pressure outside ... You cannot make a simple prohibition without considering outside circumstances (Minutes of Evidence, PP XXIX:733).

Their own experience had told them that legislative intervention could only deal with a limited number of the problems, and they resorted to persuasion and education in attempts to effect change on the ground.

The inspectors provided a resource for more 'radical' approaches to health than had hitherto generally been considered. They were prepared to argue that in many cases work was a positive rather than a negative factor in health. As Hilda Martindale (1944) suggested to the Committee on Physical Deterioration:

> ...it is impossible not be impressed by the universal preference among the women for factory over domestic work, and how depressed and out of health they become if they are obliged to remain at home (Minutes of Evidence, PP XXXII:49).

They perceived home environments to be poor, and recognized the value of companionship, wages, and a social life that a factory or workplace could offer. Also, important for our purposes, was the extent to which they gave support to feminist demands for the endowment of motherhood, and they were the first to raise the question of a state-provided maternity allowance (Anderson 1922). Their sensitivity to the needs of women was evident in numerous ways too. They were concerned about the lack of women in supervisory positions in factories, about the lack of privacy women often faced, and when medical inspection of women in lead industries was introduced, they were eventually successful in their campaign to make the provision of a private room for this purpose made compulsory. Finally they were able to make known health hazards not recognized in terms of actuality or scale. Martindale (1944) cites the example of respiratory damage from asbestos spinning which was 'met in those early days with incredulity.'

Much of what has been written about the women factory inspectors is congratulatory, and contemporary supporters, feminist and non-feminist, confirmed their own sense of achievement. However given the number of inspectors and the scale of the problems they confronted, their impact must still be regarded as somewhat limited. In addition as Jones (1988) has suggested, having women in this role, along with the constraints of a legislative approach, essentially helped to maintain women's working conditions as an 'apolitical' issue.

Feminism and the health consequences of work

The debates about industrial work had from the 1830s contained a discourse about health and the particular consequences of physical labour and long hours for women. There were those who claimed women were less able to withstand factory labour and that it also had a deleterious effect on their reproductive health. There were also those who rejected such views. In fact it could be argued that the undesirable consequences were not sufficiently established to include women within early legislation (Mockett 1988). Even when women were included in 1842 with respect to underground mine work, this was as much a concern with the 'moral' issues at stake rather than health, although the reasons for the legislation should not be seen solely in these terms either (Mark-Lawson and Witz 1988). Throughout the nineteenth and into the twentieth century, neither the essence of the debate nor the conflation of health issues with moral ones changed, but a more explicit concern with the question of women in industrial work was evident. When feminists became involved in these questions, they responded to the health dimension of the debates around 'protective' legislation in much the same terms as other activists.

Both groups of feminists responded to the attempt to restrict the employment of women in pitbrow work in the 1880s and drew on health as an argument in favour of their anti-legislative position. They drew attention to pitbrow women's physical strength and their healthy state, asserting the value of outdoor work to their robust appearance compared with their mill sisters sickly faces. As the Mayoress of Wigan informed a union conference in Bristol:

> The work of these women is very healthy. I have never, even in the country, seen women looking so robust and vigorous. They have been styled 'The Colliery Amazons and Venuses', the former on account of their strength, the latter for their pleasant faces and splendid development and beautiful teeth. (*EWR* 1893:148).

Support for these views came from local physicians, and from other supporters of the women's cause (Lown 1990). However, as John (1984) has documented, some of the negative consequences for health were completely ignored, such as accidents, the effects of cold and wet weather, and heavy moving and lifting: in fact she argues feminists were guilty of a 'romanticised account of the work' (p. 151). There were already signs of the tension that would develop between middle class feminists and their working class causes, and accusations of their geographical as well as political distance from the realities of pitbrow work were made.

Until the 1880s, hours of work dominated agitation and reform outside of the attempts at total restriction in mine work, but from the 1890s there was a new focus for questions of state intervention in the 'dangerous trades'. The 'dangerous trades' signalled a move from hours and working conditions generally to identifiable health consequences arising from exposure to hazardous gases, fumes and dusts. Such illnesses as phosphorus necrosis, plumbism or lead poisoning, arsenic and mercurial poisoning, became an avenue for medical expertise to enter directly into the state's consideration of occupational ill health (Harrison 1991a). The actual consequences of working in the 'dangerous trades', awful as these were for women, essentially affected relatively few in number compared with other working conditions. At the same time they did provide dramatic and identifiable instances of morbidity and mortality directly attributable to processes of manufacture, and they raised the question of whether women were particularly at risk. The debate about women's 'susceptibility' to the effects of factory work was again to the forefront of the interventionists' agenda.

The susceptibility argument was most evident in the case of lead poisoning, with fears that lead work also had consequences for reproduction. The case for susceptibility was medically contested and clinically unproven, but this did not lessen the belief that restriction was necessary. State intervention through inquiry and legislation increasingly sought to deal with this problem, and, in the event, it led to exclusionary measures for women from some processes in the lead industries and in the potteries in 1898 and 1903. In general, however, exclusion was not the main measure adopted; rather regulation embodied ideas of prevention that emphasized fitness for work (medical inspection), cleanliness of air, work, and workers (Harrison 1989).

Feminist activism was also caught up in the furore over the 'dangerous trades', and social feminists publicized and campaigned around these trades, especially the white lead industry. While they did support regulation, they were opposed to any restrictions on women's participation, including the suggestion that married women should be prohibited. With the support of the evidence continually provided by women factory inspectors and their own investigations, they continued to press the need to include in regulation other aspects of working conditions and further industries such as laundries. Equal rights feminists still opposed to the legislative solution, had some success in limiting the scope of regulation.

The implacable opposition of equal rights feminists to legislative interference did pose some difficulties for their response to the hazards and health effects of work. The *EWR* on a number of occasions, argued that 'every employment has its illness', in this case a reference to phosphorus necrosis (*EWR* 1894:193). On health questions, as in other spheres, they thought it was for women themselves to decide if they could do the work: 'a woman could decide herself if her strength is equal to the job' (*EWR* June 1890:243). They did not deny the reality of ill health and debility, although they frequently thought the case overstated, or they argued poverty was much more important in its origins. Discussing chain-making in the context of the Lady Commissioners Reports to the Labour Commission (1893) Jessie Boucherett wrote:

> (they)... made no complaint of loss of health, which confirmed my impression that when women get plenty of good food, they can do a surprising amount of work without suffering and that half of the illness supposed to be caused by hard work is really caused by a combination of hard work and poor food (*EWR* 1894:149).

That it was not work but other aspects of women's lives that damaged their health was a recurring theme for both groups, and it was certainly accepted in official circles as well. In the official inquiry into the death of Harriet Walters, who worked as an enameller, the White Lead Committee concluded:

> Her constitution was enfeebled by her practice of walking to her work without having tasted food and working at her dangerous employment, fasting until the dinner hour (Report 1893–4, PP. XVII).

Issues of food, home environments, poverty, long and tiring journeys to work, and long hours of domestic labour were all thought to be causes of ill health in themselves, and to predispose women to the likelihood of work-caused illness. Poverty was a key factor used in the arguments by equal rights and social feminists, as well as women inspectors, against restrictive clauses. Prohibiting women from work led, it was claimed, to a greater likelihood that both women's and their families' health would be threatened by starvation.

This concern with poverty can be viewed as an underlying rationale for social feminists' activism to obtain improved wages and an end to gender-segregated jobs where women could be confined to the worst paid and most exploitative conditions. Equal rights feminists argued along similar lines: 'It is a mockery to talk of raising the standard of comfort in the home by lowering the status of women who make the home' (*EWR* April, 1891:75). There was thus some agreement that 'protective' legislation could confirm women's disadvantage rather than alleviate it.

It was not only in this respect that there was some consensus in the analysis of the relationship between health and working conditions. Both asserted that the remedies frequently embodied in factory legislation were not preventive health measures and could only fail in this respect. As Mrs Hicks, a member of the Women's Employment Defence Association argued: 'now why instead of allowing a woman to be temporarily displaced... do not people agitate for alterations in the conditions of the unhealthy trades?' (*Shafts* March 1896:81). Ada Heather Biggs called on those attending the Women's Liberal Association 'to suggest that it should be the methods of manufacture which should be altered in the dangerous trades' (*Shafts* 1897:112). Madeleine Greenwood, a supporter of legislation argued 'they should insist on employers rendering their work as innocuous as possible to make it (the potteries) and the same applies to the match trade – insist on health conditions' (*Shafts* 1897:107). A further example was provided by Gertrude Tuckwell, Secretary of the WTUL, and a member of the 1908/1909 Committee set up to investigate the effects of lead and dust on pottery workers, who refused to agree to the committee's final recommendations. In her Memorandum stating her position she concluded: 'she should have concurred had it not been that a definite alternative exists by imposing limitations on the use of material, instead of on classes of workers' (Report 1910, PP XXIX). An examination of evidence which women inspectors gave to numerous inquiries, shows that they also shared such a view, as Miss Vines in her evidence to this same committee eloquently expressed it:

> ...unless you go to the source of the evil and stop the material itself from being unhealthy and make it innocuous, you cannot really deal with the difficulty. While the use of lead still continues, I do not believe that you will, as it were sufficiently strengthen the fence at the top of the cliff so as to prevent the need of an ambulance at the bottom (Minute of Evidence, Report 1910, PP XXIX:501).

If such a consensus existed around the nature, causes and remedies of the health consequences of work for women, why have both the health dimension and the degree of 'sisterhood' remained obscured? First, despite the visibility of this aspect of women's agitation, it was constrained by concerns with 'protective' legislation. This constraint was in part of their own making, and it seems evident that the split between equal rights and social feminists was not only constructed around their views of legislation, but also a difference in their knowledge and expertise to speak about health and working conditions. Social feminism felt that their proposed remedies were based on actual experience with the realities of women's working lives. Their approach was dictated by the conditions which they had seen for themselves. Beatrice Webb, for example, had taken work as a seamstress (Caine 1985). By implication, equal rights feminists lacked knowledge and understanding and the importance of health questions were eschewed in favour of abstract principles (Feurer 1988).

Second, questions of state intervention were not just questions of interest to women. In this respect the terms of the debate were dominated by other competing interests, and men, in a context where the state itself sought to mediate and protect capitalist interests in the workplace, and patriarchal power in the workplace and family. These interests were often in conflict over women's employment. The state had its own concerns in this respect. 'Protective' legislation itself was an indicator of a changing perception of, and role for, the state as 'guardian' of the nation's health and welfare. If industrial capitalism seemed not to be concerned with the long term interests and health of labour, it was necessary for the state to intervene in areas that had previously been sacrosanct such as the family and industrial life (Langan and Schwartz 1985; Lewis 1986). As suggested earlier, the intentions and motives of the state, although difficult to establish, were not so much with the health of women *per se*, but with the health of the nation through the preservation of separate spheres and women's particular responsibility for the health of others within their domestic role. The protective principle was not about protecting the 'vulnerable' from danger, but protecting the private sphere, thus reaffirming the public domain of work as rightfully men's, and the right of men to control both. By the end of the century, the problem of working women came to be defined as a threat to the nation's health, and this was clearly articulated in the concern with and subsequent inquiry into 'physical deterioration' (Report on Physical Deterioration 1904, PP XXXII).

There were difficulties for feminist analyses of health in this context. There was little challenge to domestic ideology although there were challenges to patriarchy in feminist struggle over state intervention. Social feminists were suspicious that proposed regulations embodied a regulation of women rather than factory conditions, and equal rights feminists constantly asserted patriarchal power as the primary motive for interference.

> The struggle that is going on now in the labour world lies between the natural desire of women to have some control of their surroundings and the desire of all men to retain all within their own hands (*EWR* 1894:147).

The ideals of domesticity, femininity and women's familial roles were, in effect, not only accepted as a framework within which activism occurred; arguably these ideals were strengthened further. Equal rights feminism sought to extend the boundaries of the domestic ideal by increasing the opportunities for women's employment so that it did not encroach on men's work, and in doing so, upheld the desirability of, and necessity for, a gendered division of labour (Lown 1990). In their commitment to a reforming state, social feminism reinforced the ideology that women were defenceless and in need of 'protection' (Thom 1986). It is evident that they did not question that women, and in particular mothers, should not have to work, or that work had undesirable consequences for the quality of domestic life and labour. This was clearly seen in their specific and divergent strategies for amelioration around homework and the sweated trades. Support for the minimum wage and the Trades Boards was based not on the principle that women's wages would be improved, but that it would raise men's, thus obviating the necessity for women to work at all. The 'family wage' or the male 'breadwinner norm' (Seecombe 1986) had become an established plank of socialist class politics and women deferred to it. Interestingly, the problems of single women were rarely discussed although the large numbers of women without the possibility of male economic support were evident in the sweated trades as elsewhere. The Women's Labour League (WLL) by 1900, had declared itself opposed to the employment of mothers with young children, and in arguing for her licensing proposal to deal with the sweated trades, Margaret MacDonald thought it might ensure 'the woman of the house used a little soap and water and made her beds each morning' (cited in Mappen 1986:247). Only in the FWG does there seem to be a clear rejection of 'a parasitic relation of women and men' and women's 'enslavement in the economy and family', but their arguments for the economic independence of women remained largely theoretical (Dyhouse 1989).

We must, however, appreciate that feminism did seek some refinements to the narrow proscriptive roles of domestic ideology: women could not fulfil their 'responsibilities' within the private sphere alone, and questions of the family were also no longer solely their responsibility. Activism around working conditions and questions of state intervention thus paved the way for further demands that health and welfare were matters for the public domain. It is also necessary to ask what would have been the practicality of a politics which espoused options for women outside of the family context? (Nicholson 1986). This seemingly conservative and negative response, as it has sometimes been viewed, might instead become 'cogent as political practice' (Levine 1988) given the reality of women's lives and the value that both middle class and working class women attached to family life (Ross 1986). Equally, issues of dependency and economic insecurity also loomed large within the Victorian family (Dyhouse 1989).

Finally, even without these constraints, it is doubtful if harnessing an analysis of the health consequences of work would have been desirable in terms of their own political priorities. In this, both social and equal rights feminists undermined the possibility of unity because other goals were uppermost. Their fundamental divergence on state interference prevented a dialogue on health and work either outside of, or as part of, these political considerations.

Working women, legislation and health

It is difficult to provide anything other than a somewhat sketchy assessment of what working women themselves thought of attempts to restrict their labour, and their views on health and work, although we must be careful not to neglect sources that may render their views more visible (Harrison 1991b). Supporters of the divergent lines of argument could always find working women who would 'testify' in ways that supported their particular point of view. Equal rights feminists had support from pitbrow women in their campaign on this particular issue, and women chain-makers had been seen on TUC platforms. There is evidence to suggest that the WTUL were more successful in recruiting women to their cause than equal rights feminists in the 1890s. For example, the latter had been active in campaigns not to extend legislation to laundries, while social feminists had urged something be done about the particularly long hours and poor conditions. In 1891 the WTUL organized a mass rally of laundresses in Hyde Park and canvassed their opinion on legislation, in which 65,939 out of 67,000 supported protection. On numerous issues, equal rights feminists chose to present canvases of employers rather than women, on the grounds that this demonstrated the effects of restricting women's hours on job opportunities. (This was certainly evident in the various attempts to limit hours in shops.) Jessie Boucherett in a comment on Clara Collet's Reports to the Labour Commission on shop assistants noted: 'it was difficult to get female assistants to complain and shows that they are not anxious for legislation' (*EWR* 1894:79). Aside from the faulty logic here, this comment belies the extent to which women did complain about their conditions. Their involvement in formal organizations was limited, but they did use these to channel grievances as the example above indicates, and the use made of the women's inspectorate was also considerable. Martindale (1944) reports that within one year of her arrival in Ireland, the number of workers complaints had risen to 300 of which one-third came from individual women. These largely anonymous individual letters, such as the one reproduced below, testify to the degree of powerlessness and fear of intimidation women experienced.

> Madam. It would do you and the poor workers of this town of B—— good if you would kindly give us a call unawares and see for yourself the awful black holes of workrooms we have to try and work in with scarcely any light the very luk of a dungeon would set one blind to say nothing of working in it.
> When you come you can look minutely into all and try and remedy all for us poor workers.
> Please say nothing when coming about receiving this letter but act upon its contents and do for us what we need in the way of proper light and ventilation.
>
> Most respectfully yours
> A Poor Worker
>
> (Martindale 1944:95)

She also reports an occasion when a deputation of eighty 'marched out of their factory in wrath and came straight to my office in order to pour out their grievances' (ibid:91).

It does seem that women could identify their grievances about working conditions and were aware of the consequences for their health. At the same time, in many public forums, they presented a view either that the work was not dangerous, or, consistent with an ideology of individual responsibility, attributed their own 'good fortune' to the fact they took good care of themselves. Such views can be found in *Minutes of Evidence to Committees of Inquiry* and should therefore be interpreted with caution, since their public nature as well as the questioning itself would have determined answers given. An ambivalence about health consequences has to be seen in the context of work as a strategy for women in their struggle with daily existence. In this respect, we also find an ambivalence toward 'protective' legislation, and the two would have become interlinked. There were many examples in the 'dangerous trades' of women changing work to avoid medical detection and then suspension. Women unionists could cite examples of where complaint often led to women losing their jobs.

We can find evidence of women's support for the social feminist case that the Factory Acts had brought positive benefits. In his survey of *Women in the Printing Trades* (1904), Ramsay MacDonald pursued this line of questioning and found them in favour, with some newer employees regretting the lack of the overtime option. These women had observed that jobs had not been threatened as a consequence. For most working women this was probably not the case. It was not just equal rights feminists who observed that many working women were opposed to legislative restriction. Social feminists, such as Clementina Black, recognized that due to simple fear of survival many women were highly suspicious of legislative protection, and Anna Martin who had considerable knowledge of working women in London noted:

> ...they know from their own experience the wholesale ruin that would result, under the present industrial system, from the passing of such a law ... the women are appalled at the idea of their liberty of action in this matter being forcibly taken away from them (cited in Dyhouse 1989:91).

Rose Squire, an inspector, had observed that by the early twentieth century, women seemed to be impatient of restriction unless shared with men. This reflects the increasing involvement of social feminism with issues of class as well as gender. We should not infer, however, that this led to any lessening of conflict with male trade unionists over 'protective' legislation. Under questioning, to the 1908/9 committee on the potteries, male trade union leaders conceded that the 'representative' views of their unions in favour of certain restrictions did not extend to the majority of their women members. Ultimately the views women had or expressed would be influenced by labour market opportunities and conditions, the extent of unionism, the realities of their own and their families economic circumstances, and therefore the meaning of work for themselves. A concern with one's own personal health was too often a luxury that could not be afforded. Women took casual, unskilled and highly dangerous work for slightly higher wages, and worked in sweated workshops and took work home for pittance wages, in an attempt to keep their families fed. Such a reality was described by Lydia Vaughan, 'a working woman'.

> In the East End of London, ... who can tell better than I what the lives of the majority of working men's wives are? The constant moiling and toiling, the dread of debt and sickness, the constant strains to make ends meet by making 20 shillings go as far as 25 shillings. How can such a woman spare time or thought beyond? (*Shafts* Dec. 3, 1892:74).

Conclusion

The focus of this chapter on feminist activism around working conditions has inevitably had to consider the health dimension within the central concern feminism had with 'protective' legislation. Working conditions and the attempts by the state to interfere directly in women's work became an important focus for feminist organizing. It was their response to this vital question of state intervention which led to division and dissent, precluding unity in political analysis and strategy on some aspects of health, the family and working lives. The state continued to pursue an analysis of the problem and its solution in protective remedies that were ineffectual in dealing with health consequences. Regulation also failed to achieve patriarchal aims of returning women to the domestic sphere.

Feminist priorities are comprehensible within the particular historical circumstances in which a feminist politics had to operate. At this time, health had few institutional bases which might have allowed women's activism on these matters to focus. Work, family life and suffrage, on the other hand, clearly articulated Victorian women's powerless position and their specific grievances within the public domain.

Finally, it would be a mistake to view the lack of an explicitly health-led campaign as resulting in a failure to provide remedy. In some respects it was limited, but we should remember that women's health states are related to a complex set of circumstances in their lives and not just to 'disease'. The feminist campaigns were all directed at women's powerlessness, and along with questions of income, maternity support, and improved sanitation, feminist activism, divided or not, was important in seeking improvements in women's health.

Notes

1. In a recent paper (Harrison 1991b), I have suggested that there may be more sources which we have neglected, which enable us to gain access to working class and poor women's subjectivity and accounts of experience.
2. The Women's Provident and Protective League (WPPL) was formed in the 1870s along with the Bristol based Women's Trade Union Association (WTUA).
3. Emma Paterson, the WPPL president, died in 1886, and although the change in leadership was not responsible for the shift in social feminist thinking, it no doubt facilitated it. The WPPL became the Women's Trade Union and Provident League in 1889, and eventually dropped the provident in 1891 to become the Women's Trade Union League (WTUL).
4. I say this because there is no mention of them in either accounts of various aspects of 'first-wave' feminism or in dictionaries of feminism (Banks 1985). This was probably due to their official position and lack of direct involvement or leadership in the major feminist struggles such as suffrage. However, a case can be made for their feminist credentials, despite the above definitional limitations. Many of the inspectors in the 1890s and early twentieth century, certainly espoused women's special virtues, their claim to the public domain, the value of women's organizations to name some, and were active supporters of both social feminist campaigns and suffrage.
5. For example, May Abraham, appointed as one of the four Assistant Lady Commissioners on the Labour Commission, and subsequently as one of the first two women factory inspectors, previously acted as secretary to Lady Dilke, a leader within the WTUL, in which Abraham was also active. A later secretary and president of the WTUL, Gertrude Tuckwell, was a niece of Lord Dilke and shared a house with May Abraham until the latter married in 1896. Both Lady Dilke and May Abraham (later Tenant) married radical MPs who supported many of their causes.

References

Anderson, A. (1922), *Women in the Factory: An Administrative Adventure*, London: John Murray.

Annual Reports of Her/His Majesty's Chief Inspectors for Factories 1880–1914, London.

Annual Reports of Her/His Majesty's Women Inspectors of Factories, 1894–1914–16, London.

Arlidge, J. (1892), *The Hygiene, Diseases and Mortality of Occupations*, London: Percival.

Banks, O. (1981), *Faces of Feminism: A Study of Feminism as a Social Movement*, Oxford: Martin Robertson.

Banks, O. (1985), *The Biographical Dictionary of British Feminists, Vol. 1800–1930*, Brighton: Wheatsheaf Books.

Boucherett, J. and Blackburn, H. (1896), *The Condition of Working Women and the Factory Acts*, London: Elliot Stock.

Caine, B. (1985), 'Beatrice Webb and the "Woman Question"', *History Workshop Journal*, **15**:25–42.
Dyhouse, C. (1989), *Feminism and the Family in England 1880–1939*, Oxford: Basil Blackwell.
English Woman's Journal and *English Woman's Review*, (various issues).
Feurer, R. (1988), 'The meaning of "sisterhood": the British women's movement and protective labour legislation 1870–1900', *Victorian Studies*, **31**:233–260.
Harding, S. (ed.) (1987), *Feminism and Methodology*, Milton Keynes: Open University Press.
Harrison, B. (1989), '"Some of them gets lead poisoned": occupational lead exposure in women 1880–1914', *Social History of Medicine*, **2**:171–195.
Harrison, B. (1990), 'Suffer the working day: women in the "dangerous trades"', *Women's Studies International Forum*, **13**:79–90.
Harrison, B. (1991a), 'Women's health or social control: the role of the medical profession in relation to factory legislation in late nineteenth century Britain', *Sociology of Health and Illness*, **13**:469–491.
Harrison, B. (1991b), 'Speaking for themselves: women's accounts of health and work in late nineteenth early twentieth century Britain', paper presented at the BSA Medical Sociology Conference, University of York, September.
Harrison, B. and Mockett, H. (1990), 'Women in the factory: the state and factory legislation in nineteenth century Britain', in Jamieson, L. and Corr, H. (eds), *State, Private Life and Political Change*, London: Macmillan.
Hutchins, B. (1915), *Women in Modern Industry*, London: G. Bell and Sons.
John, A.V. (1984), *By the Sweat of their Brow: Women in Victorian Coalmining*, London: Routledge and Kegan Paul.
Jones, H. (1988), 'Women health workers: the case of the first women factory inspectors in Britain', *Social History of Medicine*, **1**:165–181.
Lambertz, J. (1985), 'Sexual harassment in the nineteenth century English cotton industry', *History Workshop Journal*, **19**:29–63.
Langan, M. and Schwartz B. (eds) (1985), *Crises in the British State 1880–1930*, London: Hutchison.
Levine, P. (1988), *Victorian Feminism 1850–1900*, London: Hutchison Education.
Lewis, J. (1986), 'The working class wife and mother and state intervention 1870–1918', in Lewis, J. (ed.) *Labour and Love: Women's Experience of Home and Family 1850–1940*, Oxford: Basil Blackwell.
Liddington, J. and Norris, J. (1978), *One Hand Tied Behind Us*, London: Virago.
Liddington, J. (1979), 'Women cotton workers and the suffrage campaign: the radical suffragists in Lancashire 1893–1914', in Burman, S. (ed.), *Fit Work for Women*, London: Croom Helm.
Lown, J. (1990), *Women and Industrialisation: Gender at Work in Nineteenth Century England*, Cambridge: Polity Press.
MacDonald, J.R. (1904), *Women in the Printing Trades*, London: P.S. King.
McFeely, M.D. (1988), *Lady Inspectors: The Campaign for a Better Workplace 1893–1921*, Oxford: Basil Blackwell.
Mappen, E. (1985), *Helping Women at Work: The Women's Industrial Council 1889–1914*, London: Hutchison.
Mappen, E. (1986), 'Strategists for change: social feminist approaches to the

problems of women's work', in John, A.V. (ed.), *Unequal Opportunities: Women's Employment in England 1800–1918*, Oxford: Basil Blackwell.
Mark-Lawson, J. and Witz, A. (1988), 'From "family labour" to "family wage"?: the case of women's labour in nineteenth century coalmining', *Social History*, **13**:151–174.
Martindale, H. (1944), *Women Servants of the State, 1870–1938*, London: Allen and Unwin.
Mitchell, J. and Oakley, A. (1986), *What is Feminism?*, Oxford: Basil Blackwell.
Mockett, H. (1988), 'A danger to the state? Women and factory legislation 1830–1850', paper presented to BSA Annual Conference on Sociology and History, Edinburgh.
Morris, J. (1986), *Women in the Sweated Trades*, London: Avebury.
Murray, J.H. and Clarke, A.H. (1985), *The English Women's Review of Social and Industrial Questions: An Index*, New York: Garland.
Nicholson, L. (1986), *Gender and History: The Limits of Social Theory in the Age of the Family*, New York: Columbia University Press.
Oliver, T. (ed.) (1902), *Dangerous Trades: The History, Social and Legal Aspects of Industrial Occupations affecting Health by a Number of Experts*, London: John Murray.
Public Records Office, Home Office Files HO45/9848/B12393; HO45/9899/B18946; HO45/B11137/; HO45/9933/B26610.
Ramazanoglu, C. (1989), *Feminism and the Contradiction of Oppression*, London: Routledge.
Report of the Departmental Committee on the Various Lead Industries, (1893–4), PP XVII.
Report of Her Majesty's Principal Secretary of State for the Home Department on the Conditions of Labour in the Potteries the Injurous Effects upon Health of the Workpeople and the Proposed Remedies (Also known as the Potteries Committee of Inquiry 1893–4), PP XVII.
Report on a Committee to Inquire into the Working of the Cotton Cloth Factories Act 1889 (1897), PP XVII.
Report of Her Majesty's Principal Secretary of State for the Home Department on the Employment of Compounds of Lead in the Manufacture of Pottery, their Influence on the Health of the Workpeople, with Suggestions as to the Means which Might be Adopted to Counteract their Evil Effects, (1899), PP XII.
Reports to the Secretary of State for the Home Department on the Use of Phosphorous in the Manufacture of Lucifer Matches, (1899), PP XII.
Report of the Interdepartmental Committee on Physical Deterioration and Evidence (1904), PP XXXII.
Report of the Departmental Committee Appointed to Inquire into the Dangers Attendant on the Use of Lead, and the Danger or Injury to Health Arising from Dust and other Causes in the Manufacture of Earthenware and China and the Processes Incidental thereto in the Making of Lithographic Transfers, (1910) and Minutes of Evidence PP XXIX.
Riley, D. (1988), *'Am I That Name?': Feminism and the Category of 'Women' in History*, London: Macmillan.
Ross, E. (1986), 'Labour and love: rediscovering London's working class moth-

ers', in Lewis, J. (ed.), *Labour and Love: Women's Experience of Home and Family 1850–1949*, Oxford: Basil Blackwell.
Rowbotham, S. (1977), *Hidden from History: 300 Years of Women's Oppression and How to Fight it*, London: Pluto.
Royal Commission on Labour (1893–4), *The Reports of the Assistant Lady Commissioners on the Conditions of Work of Women and Girls in England, Wales, Scotland and Ireland*, PP XXXVII.
Scott, J.W. (1987), 'On language, gender and working class history', *International Labor and Working Class History*, **31**:1–13.
Scott, J.W. (1988), 'The problem of invisibility', in Kleinberg, S.J. (ed.), *Retrieving Women's History: Changing Perceptions of the Role of Women in Politics and Society*, Oxford: Berg.
Seecombe, W. (1986), 'Patriarchy stabilised: the construction of the male breadwinner norm in nineteenth century Britain', *Social History*, **11**:53–76.
Shafts, (various issues).
Squire, R. (1927), *Thirty Years in the Public Service: An Industrial Retrospect*, London: Nisbet and Co.
Stanley, L. (1990), 'Rediscovering women in history from feminist deconstructionism', *Women's Studies International Forum*, **13**:151–158.
The Gertrude Tuckwell Collection, TUC Library, Congress House London.
Thom, D. (1986), 'The bundle of sticks: women trade unionists and collective organisation before 1918', in John, A.V. (ed.), *Unequal Opportunities: Women's Employment in England 1900–1918*, Oxford: Basil Blackwell.
Tuckwell, G.M. *et al.* (1908), *Women in Industry*, London: Duckworth.
Walby, S. (1986), *Patriarchy at Work: Patriarchal and Capitalist Relations in Employment*, Oxford: Polity Press.
Walby, S. (1990), 'From private to public patriarchy: the periodisation of British history', *Women's Studies International Forum*, **13**:91–104.
Webb, B. (1902), *Women and the Factory Acts*, Fabian Tract No. 67, also reprinted in Webb, S. and B. (eds) *Problems of Modern Industry*, London: Longmans Green.
Wohl, A. (1983), *Endangered Lives: Public Health in Victorian England*, London: J.M. Dent and Sons.

6 Conditions of formal and domestic labour

Toward an integrated framework for the analysis of gender and social class inequalities in health

Jennie Popay and Mel Bartley

> What constitutes the alienation of labour? First that work is external to the worker...consequently, he (*sic*) does not fulfil himself in his work...has a feeling of misery rather than well-being, does not develop freely his mental and physical energies, but is physically exhausted and mentally debased.
>
> (Karl Marx, quoted in Bottomore, 1963)

Introduction

Since Marx wrote of the process of alienation, an impressive array of evidence has been amassed on the adverse effect of poor material and psychosocial conditions of labour for the physical and mental health of paid workers. In this chapter, we attempt to draw on this literature to develop an integrated framework for analysing gender and social class inequalities in health. To avoid confusion we must stress at the outset that we are not centrally concerned with the sociological debates on the need for an integration of class and gender analyses. According to Dex, as researchers who want to use social class categories to explain other behaviours, we are 'located outside the realm of pure sociological theory' (Dex 1985, p. 152). We seek to better understand the way in which patterns of ill health associated with social class interact with those associated with gender. However, and to return to Dex, we do not intend to 'continue to use but complain about official social class categories'. Nor do we wish to accept crude measures of gender – basically sex. Rather, we hope that through a reconceptualization of conditions of labour it may be possible – at least in the health field – to bridge the class/gender divide evident in much previous research on inequalities in health.

We begin by briefly reviewing the literature on the relationship between conditions of labour and the experience of health and illness. We will argue that, although women's and men's experiences are presented as fundamentally different in this work, it does provide insights into how a more integrated conceptualization might begin. Second, we describe our attempt to operationalize new concepts of labour conditions, which can be used to compare the relationship between different work roles and health and illness, regardless of sex, and across social class. Third, we present some provisional findings using these measures to address three questions: *How do our new measures perform, in terms of their predictive power compared to traditional ways of measuring domestic and formal working conditions?; What is the relative importance of domestic and formal labour conditions in shaping the experience of health and illness amongst women and men?; In what ways, if any, do conditions of labour in one sphere of labour interact with those in another to shape women's and men's experiences of health and illness?*

Review of the literature

In recent years, there has been a surge of interest amongst researchers, policy makers and health care professionals, in the health experience of people in different social classes (Whitehead 1987; Davey-Smith *et al.* 1990). To a lesser extent, though still notable, there has also been a growth of interest in the different health experiences of women and men (Verbrugge 1989; Karasek *et al.* 1983; Verbrugge *et al.* 1987; Silman 1987; Koskenvuo *et al.* 1986; Celantano *et al.* 1990). Both of these fields of work contain explicit and implicit reference to conditions of labour. There are, however, important differences between research concerned with social class and that concerned with gender-related inequalities in health and particularly there are fundamental differences in the way conditions of labour have been conceptualized.

Research on social class has been focused above all on differential mortality experience – primarily of men (Wilkinson 1986). The aetiological significance of people's public lives in paid work and the material conditions in which they live and work have been an important and influential focus in this research. This is reflected in the pervasive use of occupation as a measure of social class, in studies of specific occupational hazards and in work on the health consequences of poor housing and low income (Fox and Goldblatt 1982; Martin *et al.* 1987; Marmot *et al.* 1984; Wilkinson 1990). More recently, considerable research effort, in Europe at least, has been directed at the health effects of the psychosocial conditions of paid labour, though again this work has focused primarily on men's experiences

(Karasek *et al.* 1981; Marmot *et al.* 1984, 1987; Cooper and Smith 1985; Baruch *et al.* 1987).

Research on gender inequalities in health has also paid some attention to mortality patterns. In the wealthier Western nations at least, the mortality rates amongst men are strikingly higher than amongst women. So much so in fact, that at different times and in all industrialized countries, men's life expectancy is consistently found to be lower, by between five and ten years, than women's. In contrast, however, women experience a great deal more non-life threatening illness than men and research on gender inequalities in health has focused primarily on this morbidity differential. Also, in contrast to the research on class inequalities in health, the major focus of research on gender differences in ill health has been the aetiological significance of the psychosocial conditions of domestic labour.

These divisions in research on social class and gender inequalities in health, have had serious consequences for our understanding of aetiology in relation to women's and men's experience of health and illness. They have resulted, for example, in a neglect of the private lives of men, although as already noted, increasing attention is being paid to the psychosocial dimensions of men's public lives. In contrast, women's private lives, and their world of domestic labour, have been the focus of considerable attention, but the material aspects of these experiences have received little sustained study. Additionally, whilst their involvement in paid work has received considerable attention, it is employment status *per se* which is the focus, rather than the conditions of paid labour (Bartley *et al.* 1992).

Research on social class inequalities powerfully illustrates these limitations. For example, there is a consistent failure to use measures sensitive to material disadvantage amongst women. First, most occupationally based measures of social class are constructed from a classification of occupations which are predominantly male and therefore insensitive to the differences between women's occupations. Though the classification system developed by Roberts (1987) goes some way to remedy this limitation, it is not widely used whilst the revised occupational classification to be used in future for the RGSC (the Registrar General's Social Class Classification) appears to represent only a marginal improvement in this particular sphere. Second, commonly used measures of social class cannot locate an increasing number of people, many of whom are women, who depend in the long term on the social security system or on a partner for their financial support. Third, they are a very crude measure of individual living standards, unable to deal with the possibility of unequal access to resources within households. Finally, research focusing on the public world of paid employment does not and cannot offer insights into the health implications of conditions in the private world of the family. As Townsend (1990) has recently argued, 'occupational class cannot be social class' and nowhere is this more profoundly apparent than in relation to the experience of women.

Unfortunately, this bias in research on social class inequalities in health is not compensated for by research on gender inequalities. Here, the focus has been on women's social role in the family and on the different socialization of women compared to men. Together, it is argued that these mean that women are readier than men to report sickness or to adopt the sick role. Neglected is the possibility that women may really be sicker than men and that the demands of their domestic labour and the material conditions they labour in, may make a major contribution to their experience of ill health (Gove and Hughes 1981).

The notion of treating domestic activity as work has, of course, a long and more or less respectable history within the social sciences. Ann Oakley (1974), for example, described the housewife as:

> a woman involved in an occupation, which has all the characteristics of other work roles except one – it is unpaid.

Oakley and others have detailed many of the characteristics of this 'occupation', that it is unstructured, unrewarding, invisible, often isolated and contains a high degree of 'emotional work' – work that is necessary to make other people feel good (Graham 1983; Finch and Groves 1983; Boulton 1986). It could be argued that all women share these aspects of the experience of domestic labour, albeit to a greater or lesser extent. However, the fact that, like paid work, the experience of domestic labour divides women by social class has been neglected within recent feminist scholarship, with honourable exceptions (Graham 1985). Interestingly, this was less so in the past, when the demands of domestic labour for poor women were perhaps more visible (Spring-Rice Davies 1939). So little contemporary attention has been paid to this area that we know very little about how class divisions are experienced by women in the late twentieth century. However, it should be obvious that the nature of domestic labour will vary depending on the physical and material circumstances in which such labour is undertaken.

Towards an integrated theory of labour conditions and the health of women and men

Despite the limitations and gender blindness of existing research on the health implications of formal labour it does provide a base line from which to begin to reconceptualize labour conditions to take account of women's unpaid work. This reconceptualization is, in turn, a pre-requisite for the development of an integrated theory of the relationship between social class, gender and health. In order to develop a unified concept of labour conditions, we have drawn ideas from a number of different spheres of work notably that of Townsend and Karasek (Townsend 1979; Karasek

1979, 1981, 1989). It is our view that Townsend's work on the concept of 'occupational deprivation' is amongst the most innovative of recent contributions to research on the relationship between formal labour conditions and social class inequalities in health. He is concerned, in particular, with material conditions of labour and the index he has been constructing has four main dimensions: income from work; the relative security of the job; the conditions and amenities at work; and the fringe benefits attaching to the job. Transferring elements of this index to the domestic sphere presents formidable difficulties. However, it also raises important questions about the way in which the concept is being elaborated and operationalized in the formal labour market. Take income, for example, is it possible to transfer a concept of income from employment into the domestic sphere? One could simply argue that those involved in the domestic sphere do not 'earn' an income. But this is not strictly accurate. What of child benefit, housekeeping allowances, state benefits to women not in employment and to foster parents? Exploring this issue forces one to consider exactly what it is about income that is important in relation to health inequalities. Access to resources for personal consumption or for collective consumption? Access to a means of control and a source of power? Such questions are being addressed by some researchers in the field of gender inequalities in health and obviously have implications too for the measures of income used in relation to the formal labour market (Rosenfeld 1989).

Perhaps the most straightforward example of the way in which a concept of occupational deprivation might be extended to the domestic sphere is provided by Townsend's measures of hazards at work. For instance, the experience of pollution, damp, noise, overcrowded and unsafe conditions, are readily seen to be equally applicable to both the domestic and the formal labour sectors.

In contrast to Townsend, Karasek and his colleagues have been concerned to develop measures of the psychosocial conditions of paid labour, rather than material conditions – a focus evident in this country in the work of Marmot and colleagues on the Whitehall study (Marmot *et al.* 1984). Karasek *et al.* have refined the notoriously elusive concept of stress into two dimensions: job demand and job decision latitude. *Job demand*, according to these researchers, refers to the psychosocial pressures involved in different forms of paid work, whilst *job decision latitude* is the scope offered in a particular job for the individual to exercise autonomy and achieve self-actualization, as well as to adapt the pace of work according to their own discretion. Job demand has been operationalized in terms of such features as the length of the working day, machine pacing of work and unspecified 'problems' with superiors or workmates. Job decision latitude has been operationalized in terms of whether or not workers are able to make or receive private phone calls or leave work for short periods on private business.

One has only to itemize the questionnaire items that have been used in the literature to realize how difficult it is to devise appropriate measures of the wide variety of psycho-social conditions under which people labour, even in the formal sector of the economy. It is however, possible to see how concepts of job demand and job decision latitude, might be applied in theory at least in the domestic sphere. For instance, one dimension of demand explored by Karasek *et al.* (1981) is the extent to which a job is hectic. What could be more hectic than the demands of say, two children under five, combined with the demands of a dependent elderly person, perhaps in the context of an unhelpful partner and the absence of convenient, safe play space and working domestic appliances? This example illustrates both how the concept might be transferred to the domestic sphere and also how it might be operationalized. Job decision latitude is similarly transferable. Take, for example, time off work for personal reasons. Once again, it takes only a little imagination, at least for women, to see how little

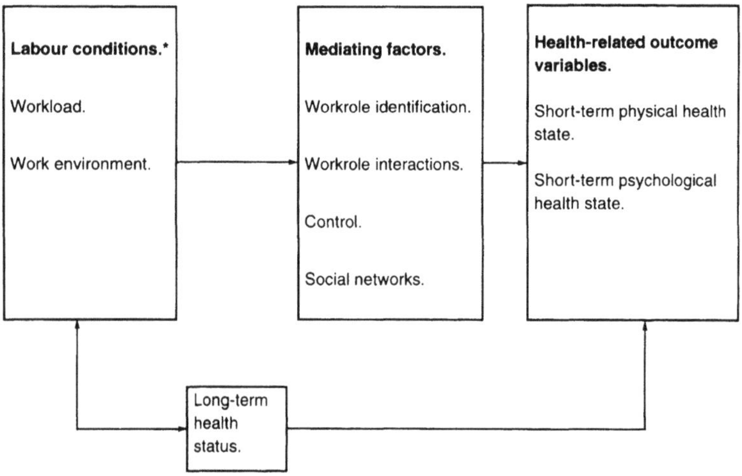

Note: *Both of these have material and psychosocial dimensions and both have positive and negative aspects.

Figure 1 A conceptual model of an integrated approach to class and gender inequalities in health

latitude there will be for doing this, even for thinking one's own thoughts, if you were in the domestic situation described above.

Drawing on the literature described here and elsewhere, we have developed the following conceptual model to help us to untangle the interactions between gender and social class inequalities in health (Figure 1). The model, has four major dimensions: *labour conditions, mediating factors, long term illness* (which we include separately as long-term health status, in order to take account of the possibility of health-related selection into particular social positions) and *health-related outcomes*. Operationalizing these concepts in a measurable form using existing data sets, was quite another matter.

From concepts to measures: the limits of secondary analysis

The research reported on here was part of a larger study based on the secondary analysis of three existing data sets: the General Household Survey (GHS), the Health and Lifestyles Survey (HALS) and the London Standard of Living Survey (LSLS). At an early stage we abandoned the notion of combining information from the three surveys in one analysis and sought to answer different questions with different data sets. In any one exercise, however, we were able only to produce a partial set of measures.

In this chapter we present some of the analysis of the London Standard of Living Survey data. In the remainder of this section we focus on the measures of labour conditions we have developed from the LSLS data set and the health-related measures we have used. In the next section we present some provisional findings relating to the three questions identified earlier. Our work with the other data sets is discussed elsewhere (Popay, Bartley and Owen 1992; Bartley, Popay and Plewis 1992; Bartley and Owen 1991 unpublished; Popay and Bartley 1989).

Measuring conditions of labour

The London Standard of Living Survey was conducted in 1985/86 and collected data from 1,716 households and 2,703 adults representative of the Greater London population. A detailed account of the methodology is reported elsewhere (Owen 1987). The analysis presented here has been carried out only on those sample members aged between 18 and 64 who could be allocated a score on all the relevant variables needed to construct our labour condition measures: 943 women and 828 men.

To return to the theoretical model in Figure 1 we began with three main dimensions: labour conditions, mediating factors and health-related outcomes. The analysis reported here does not incorporate any of the mediating factors shown in the theoretical model. Within labour conditions we had identified two separate aspects, workload and work environment relevant to both domestic and paid labour. We had conceptualized both workload and work environment as having physical and psychosocial dimensions, which in some circumstances may be balanced off against one another, whilst in others, the burden could be cumulative.

The method used to construct our measures was based on techniques used in psychological measurement. An underlying concept may be operationalized in terms of a number of items which are chosen on the basis of their face validity. Any one of these will be a relatively imprecise measure but, by using a number in combination, a better estimate is achieved. Having provisionally selected items from a data set on the basis of face validity, the correlations between these is tested. In psychometrics, a high degree of correlation between items is usually required before these can be combined into a scale. Developing measures of material or psychosocial labour conditions, however, is a somewhat different matter. Sociologists would not assume that all items need be closely correlated in order to be included in a summary measure. For example, income and prestige included in measures of social class are not always highly correlated. However, if some items were negatively correlated this would indicate the need for more than one scale.

The first task we faced was to go through the LSLS data set listing existing variables or the potential for constructing variables which had some degree of face validity in relation to domestic and formal paid workload and work environment. However, in none of our data sets was there sufficient information to allow us to construct separate measures for workload and environment. We have therefore been working with combined measures of domestic and paid labour conditions. In LSLS, we were able to construct separate measures for the material and psychosocial conditions of paid labour. However, for domestic labour conditions, information on psychosocial aspects was sorely lacking, so a single measure, largely incorporating material items, was constructed.

Figure 2 shows the items included in the measure of the material conditions associated with formal paid labour. This was one of the most straightforward measures to construct as it involved combining existing variables rather than constructing new ones. However, that should not be interpreted as meaning this work was simple, as anyone who has done secondary analysis would know. Items four and five in this list, conditions and amenities at work and exposure to hazards, are themselves composite scores (see Figures 3 and 4). The items included in conditions and amenities at work were marginally different for indoor and outdoor work. Figure 5 shows the composition of the negative psychosocial conditions of formal paid labour.

Constructing the measure of domestic labour conditions was considerably more complex. This stemmed in large part from the fact that domestic

1. Subjective perception of long hours
2. Standing up for more than quarter of day
3. Regular unsocial hours
4. Conditions and amenities at work
5. Exposure to hazards

Figure 2 Material conditions of formal work

1. Tea/coffee facilities to make hot drink
2. Indoor place to eat during breaks
3. A lavatory
4. Safe place to keep coat/spare clothes
5. Safe place to keep money/valuables
6. First aid box or first aid facilities
7. Chance to make/receive at least one phone call
8. Lighting which can be increased/decreased
9. Dry/warm place to shelter

Figure 3 Conditions and amenities of outdoor work

Polluted air
Moisture/dampness
Noise
Vibration
Heavy lifting
High temperature
Low temperature
Bad lighting

Figure 4 Exposure to hazards

1. Has supervisory responsibility
2. Wish to leave job
3. Experience discrimination
4. Experience working conditions as bad for health

Figure 5 Negative psychosocial conditions of formal work

labour was not conceptualized within the LSLS in the same way as paid labour. A great deal of information was collected on the material conditions in the home and the wider environment, and this we were able to use. However, it was not always readily attributable to the experience of any one individual within a household. Additionally, some questions were simply not asked. People involved in domestic labour, for example, were not asked whether they experienced a problem with noise in the home, though anyone who has cared for squabbling children or has had to cope with the persistent crying of a young baby will realize that it can be a prominent feature of domestic labour conditions.

Our methodological coat therefore had to be cut to fit the gendered cloth with which we were working. We were brought sharply up against the constraints inherent in any attempt to use secondary data sources to move beyond traditional operationalizations associated with concepts of social class and gender. The reality is that constructions of class and gender are so embedded in the research instruments themselves that the raw data is fundamentally flawed.

That said, we do believe that we have been able to construct a measure of domestic labour conditions that goes some way to achieving our objectives. Traditionally, to the extent that research has taken account of the nature and scale of domestic labour, it has relied on number and age of children as a measurable operationalization of this. Clearly, this neglects other important aspects of the job, such as the care of elderly and/or frail relatives, for example. Additionally, these traditional approaches to the measurement of domestic labour conditions do not attempt to take account of the material environment in which the labour takes place. As Figure 6 illustrates, we have tried to address these two dimensions in our measure.

1. Age of youngest child less than 3 years
2. Number of children in the household
3. Caring for a dependent adult inside/outside the home
4. Unemployed person in the household
5. Lone parent in the household
6. Lacking essential consumer goods
7. Cannot afford convenience goods
8. Conditions and amenities in the home
9. Overcrowded conditions
10. Sharing accommodation
11. Conditions and amenities in the local area
12. Subjective perception of conditions as bad for health

Figure 6 Domestic labour conditions

Within the overall domestic labour conditions measure, there are items which themselves represent the sum of multiple indices. Lacking essential goods, for example, includes absence of any of the following for any reason: car, fridge, iron, cooker, telephone, vacuum cleaner, TV and carpets. We also distinguished between these essential items and the absence of a range of convenience goods which may make the burden of domestic labour easier but which people may choose not to own. Item 7 in Figure 6 therefore refers to the lack of one or more of the following because of lack of money: video, food mixer, dishwasher, freezer etc. The two items on conditions and amenities in the home and the local area attempt to replicate similar items included in the measure of material labour conditions in the formal sphere and the details of these are shown in Figures 7 and 8.

No central heating
No indoor wc/bath
No electricity
Most rooms unheated in winter
Damp housing
Insect infested housing
Housing in poor external repair

Figure 7 Conditions and amenities in the home

No open space
No recreational facilities
No shops nearby
Dirty streets
No doctor or hospital nearby
No space for children to play inside
No playspace outside for children aged 5–10

Figure 8 Conditions and amenities in the local area

Once we had identified existing items with face validity, as indicators of labour conditions, correlations between items for any one measure were checked using the 'reliability' procedure in SPSS.X and by factor analysis. The items eventually included in our measures were all positively correlated and all fell within a single factor when analysed together with a larger set. Some of the original items were scored as 0,1 whilst others had a greater range. All items were therefore standardized using the 'descriptives' procedure in SPSS.X. The resulting 'Z-scores' were then summed to form a scale.

To summarize, using the London Standard of Living Survey data, we have constructed three separate measures of labour conditions with the following ranges:

Women	Formal physical conditions	0–61
	Formal psychosocial conditions	0–44
	Domestic conditions	0–55
Men	Formal physical conditions	0–60
	Formal psychosocial conditions	0–63.5
	Domestic conditions	0–63

Having done this, however, we were left with a final problem: could we take account of differential exposure to adverse working conditions? This notion has long been accorded significance in scientific work on occupational hazards and with epidemiology more generally. It is, of course, plausible that the length of time an individual is exposed to a hazard to health is likely to be a critical factor determining the scale of damage done. A senior architect exposed to the hazards of a building site for perhaps a day a week, can be expected to suffer fewer related health problems than a bricklayer. Similarly, a woman caring full time for two young children will be more likely to experience related health problems, than her partner who cares for the children for a few hours a week, albeit concentrated at the weekend. This, of course, raises the somewhat thorny issue of the double day. A woman with two young children who also has a part time paid job may have a lower exposure to the health hazards of domestic labour than a full-time housewife/mother. However, in theory at least, she may also be exposed to adverse labour conditions in the formal sector. Alternatively, the benefits of one type of labour may compensate for the demands of the other.

However, despite the theoretical importance of exposure times, we were not able to incorporate this into the analysis presented in this paper. Whilst the LSLS does contain detailed estimates of the amount of time spent on different aspects of domestic labour, including housework, caring for children and caring for other dependents, and information on hours of formal paid labour, the latter was missing for around a quarter of our sample. Whilst it is technically possible to derive average exposure times, arriving at an acceptable basis for doing this is problematic. Additionally, the kind of health-related outcome measure used in our analysis made it difficult to incorporate exposure times. Hours of work, either formal or domestic, may have a different relationship to measures of health which include limitation of activity, than to measures such as symptom checklists. For example, a man working long hours is probably younger than one who is not. He may also be 'selected' into such a position by good health. Likewise, the majority of women working long hours in the home are those with young children who are therefore younger women. One would therefore need to compare the results of analysis using different kinds of outcome measures but the LSLS data set does not contain a symptom checklist. We hope to address this issue in further work.

Measuring ill-health

In our previous work we have shown the importance of looking separately at three different dimensions of ill-health: long-term health status and short-term physical and psychological health state (Blaxter 1990; Bartley *et al.* 1992). Within the LSLS data set, we have been able to construct a measure of long-term health status – a measure attempting to identify the presence of chronic illness or disability. This has been constructed from the answers to two questions. The first asks about the experience of 'regular or lasting trouble which prevent you from doing the things you might expect to do at your age', in relation to the items shown in Figure 9. The second question focuses on whether and in what way a problem limits activity or social interaction. This measure of long-term health status is incorporated into our theoretical and analytical model as a factor potentially confounding the relationship between labour conditions and short-term health outcomes.

Back or spine
Legs or feet
Joints
Arms or hands
Chest or lungs
Eyesight
Hearing
Speech
Nerves
Fits and blackouts

Figure 9 Lasting/regular health problems included in the London Standard of Living Survey

The other health-related measures available in LSLS were extremely limited. There were two measures available to us: a measure of recent restricted illness and a measure of perceptions of health in general over a 12 month period. Neither the recent restricting illness measure, nor the measure of global health were able to be separated into the physical and psychological components of health and illness. The analysis presented in this paper uses only the recent restricted illness measure as an outcome variable. It is important to recognize that this type of measure is notoriously confounded with illness behaviour and therefore with workroles themselves, as we discuss when interpreting our findings.

Other variables included in the analysis

In addition to our constructed measures of working conditions and the health-related variables discussed above, our analysis includes two more traditional measures of labour conditions: occupational social class and employment status. Registrar general occupational social class was available in the LSLS and we used three categories for women (professional/managerial, clerical and manual) and four categories for men (professional/managerial, skilled non-manual, skilled manual and semi/unskilled manual). In relation to employment status, the categories used for men and women also varied: for women we used full-time housework, part-time employed and full-time employed, whilst for men we used unemployed and employed.

Statistical analysis

As we noted at the beginning of this paper our analysis has been concerned with exploring three issues: the relationship between our new measures of labour conditions and the experience of ill-health; the relative importance of formal and domestic labour conditions in shaping individual experiences of ill-health; and the way in which labour conditions in the domestic and formal spheres interact. The measures we have been developing, aim to make women's and men's experiences comparable by, for example, avoiding the use of categories such as 'occupational class' and 'full-time versus part-time' employment, which have totally different meanings when applied to women and men.

In order to address these issues we used a proportional odds modelling technique. The assumptions underlying this technique are that the outcome variable is ordered and that a one unit change in the explanatory variables produces an equal change in the risk of moving between each category of the outcome variable. It should be stressed that it is not the purpose of logistic regression as used here to test either goodness-of-fit or to explain the variation in the data overall. We are not concerned with the overall power of the model. Rather, this approach allowed us to consider the relative power of individual factors in explaining the experience of recent restricting illness and to estimate the relative risk of experiencing recent restricting illness associated with each of our factors.

Because our labour conditions scores are continuous scores with quite extensive ranges, the effect of a one unit change in these scores on the health outcome measure will inevitably be small. In order to make meaningful comparisons with the risk associated with a unit change in the traditional measures of occupational social class and employment status, which have a much smaller number of units, the risk associated with a one unit change in the new measures has been multiplied up to show the relative risk associated with the top of the range of each score, compared to the bottom of the range.

Findings

Our first step was to apply the traditional measures of labour conditions – occupational social class and employment status – together with our measure of domestic labour conditions and existing long-term health status within a model for women only. The results are shown in Table 1. As can be seen from this table, whilst long-term health status and domestic conditions made a significant contribution to the power of the model, occupational social class and employment status added nothing. The relative risk associated with each of the factors is also shown in Table 1 and it can be seen here that having a chronic illness makes it just over twice as likely that a woman will have had some recent illness and that this illness will have entailed some restriction of activity. In comparison, a woman with the maximum domestic conditions score has a three times greater risk of experiencing a more severe category of recent restricting illness than a woman with the lowest score, independently of long-term health status, social class and employment status. Although we had expected the effect on health of domestic conditions to be influenced by whether or not women were also in paid employment, there was no significant interaction effect in this model or indeed in any of our models.

The linear relationship evident for the relative risks associated with occupational social class are worthy of note, although these are not significant. The gradient, with a higher risk of experiencing recent illness in higher social classes, is in fact the reverse of that commonly found for mortality and chronic illness for example, and this is probably linked to the nature of the outcome measure we are using. As we have already noted, measures of illness linked to activity restriction will be confounded with role obligations and it is likely that the linear trend evident here is a function of the stronger effects of health-related selection into work in women compared to men. Only the healthiest women can be expected to remain in paid work in classes III, IV, and V.

Table 2 contains the results for a model, again focusing on women, but which included our newly constructed measures of formal physical conditions and formal psychosocial conditions, rather than occupational social class and employment status. As in the previous model, long-term health status and our domestic conditions measure contribute significantly to the model independently of each other. However, unlike class and employment status in the previous model, the two new formal conditions measures also contribute independent and significant additions to the power of this second model. The three new measures of labour conditions included in this model also increase the risk of higher levels of illness by similar amounts

Table 1 Proportional odds analysis: Women aged 18–59, conventional measures of formal labour conditions/ new domestic conditions measure

Measure	X2	df	log R	SER	Relative risk	P value
Chronic illness	23.96	1	0.7467	0.1560	+2.1	<0.01
Class						
Prof./ Managerial 1*	23.70	2	–0.1710	0.1086	1.00	–
Clerical 2	–	–	–	–	0.84	ns
Manual 3	–	–	–	–	0.71	ns
Employment status						
Housewife	24.51	4**	–	–	1.00	–
Full-time employed	–	–	0.2554	0.1842	1.29	ns
Part-time employed	–	–	0.0860	0.2152	1.09	ns
Domestic conditions	33.58	5	0.0242	0.0080	1.02 for 1 unit 3.02 from bottom to top of range	<0.05

* Class was treated as a continuous variable, class 1 (professional/managerial) is a baseline, therefore relative risks relate to the risk of experiencing more severe recent illness in clerical or manual classes compared to professional/managerial.

** Employment status was included as two dummy variables with one degree of freedom each.

Table 2 Proportional odds analysis: Women 18–59, new measures of formal physical and psychosocial labour conditions*

Measure	X2	df	log R	SER	Relative risk	P value
Chronic illness	23.96	1	0.7265	0.1519	2.07	<0.01
Formal physical conditions	31.83	2	0.0185	0.0071	1.02 for 1 unit increase in score 3.1 bottom to top of score	<0.005
Formal psychosocial conditions	35.72	3	0.0150	0.0072	1.01 for 1 unit increase 1.95 from bottom to top	<0.05
Domestic conditions	40.28	4	0.0155	0.0072	1.02 for 1 unit increase 2.35 from bottom to top	<0.05

* Range of scores on constructed measures:
Formal physical conditions 0–61.
Formal psychosocial conditions 0–44.
Domestic conditions 0–55.

per unit change in the score. The increase in risk of experiencing a more severe recent restricting illness associated with the highest score on each measure relative to the lowest score, is greatest for formal physical conditions, followed by that associated with domestic conditions and then formal psychosocial conditions. We again found no significant interaction between domestic and formal conditions. That is, for example, a woman with poor domestic conditions in a 'heavy' paid job is neither more nor less likely to experience a higher level of recent illness than one with the same domestic workload who has a lighter job, and vice versa.

Repeating the analysis for men presented us with a somewhat different picture. The results presented in Table 3 confirm the dominance of chronic illness as a factor explaining the experience of recent illness. However, they also indicate that none of the labour condition variables included in these analyses made a significant contribution to the explanatory power of the model over and above that of long-term health status, though the effect of domestic conditions was on the margins of significance. Despite the lack of significance attaching to the results, it is worth noting that the relative risk of experiencing more severe recent illness is almost three times greater amongst those men with the highest domestic conditions scores compared to those with the lowest score.

It is also of note that, although statistically insignificant, the linear trend for the relative risk associated with occupational class is in the expected direction, with the risk increasing in lower classes, in contrast to that found amongst women. The lack of a statistically significant class effect is perhaps surprising, given the enormous literature on the relationship between class and many dimensions of ill-health and mortality. However, it is likely that this is in part due to the way in which our outcome measure of recent restricting illness may be confounded with illness behaviour which is, in turn, likely to be linked to the demands of people's social roles. Certainly, results from the General Household Survey show inconsistent social class patterns for a similar measure.

The pattern of relative risks evident in relation to employment status, (again statistically insignificant) with the unemployed having an 11 per cent lower risk of experiencing more severe recent illness than the employed, is probably also due to the nature of our outcome measure. Most of the work exploring the relationship between work and health, using a measure of recent restricting illness as the health-related measure, has concentrated on women (Arber *et al.* 1985). It is therefore difficult to know whether this pattern is what one should have expected. However, it is certainly to be expected, in that unemployed men will obviously be less likely to experience 'restriction' due to illness in the form of time off work, for example. In addition, as others have shown, men perform relatively little domestic labour, even when unemployed, so that unemployed men have few domestic obligations to be restricted (Kowarzik and Popay 1989).

Table 3 Proportional odds analysis: Men aged 18–59, conventional measures of formal working conditions/ new domestic conditions measure

Measure	X2	df	log R	SER	Relative risk	P value
Chronic illness	17.14	1	0.7188	0.7139	2.05	<0.01
Class *	18.81	2	0.0370	0.0767	–	–
Prof./ Managerial 1		–			1.00	ns
Non-manual 2	–	–	–	–	1.04	ns
Skilled manual 3	–	–	–	–	1.08	ns
Semi/unskilled manual 4	–	–	–	–	1.12	ns
Employment status**	18.82	3	0.1164	0.2610	0.89	ns
Domestic conditions***	22.49	4	0.0161	0.0083	1.02 for each unit increase in score 2.76 from bottom to top of score	ns

* See note to Table 1.
** For men employment status was either employed or unemployed. The relative risk shown is unemployed relative to employed.
*** Amongst men the range on this measure was 0–63.

Table 4 Proportional odds analysis: Men aged 18–59, new measures of formal physical and psychosocial labour conditions* and domestic conditions

Measure	X2	df	log R	SER	Relative risk	P value
Chronic illness	17.14	1	0.680	0.1710	1.97	<0.01
Formal physical workload	17.32	2 –	0.0014	0.0083	1.001 for 1 unit increase in score 1.100 bottom to top of score	ns
Formal psychosocial conditions	19.32	3	0.0105	0.0080	1.01 for 1 unit increase 1.90 from bottom to top of range	ns
Domestic conditions	23.11	4	0.0154	0.0078	1.02 for 1 unit increase in score 2.57 from bottom to top of range	<0.1

* Range of scores in formal condition measures:
Physical conditions 0–60.
Psychosocial conditions 0–63.5.

The final table (Table 4) shows the results for the analysis including our newly constructed measures of formal labour conditions for men. The picture here is also different from that for women, with the new measures of formal labour conditions performing little better than the traditional measures. Here again, the effect of our domestic conditions measure on the explanatory power of the model is on the margins of significance and the relative risk of experiencing more severe recent illness associated with the highest score on this measure, is two and a half times greater than that associated with the lowest score. Though it should be remembered that the results are not statistically significant, it is of interest to note that there is virtually no difference in the relative risk of experiencing more severe recent illness amongst men with the worst and the best physical conditions in paid work. In contrast, men with the worst psychosocial conditions are almost twice as likely to experience more severe recent illness than those with the best psychosocial conditions.

Conclusions

We were concerned with three questions in this chapter. The first was the comparison between the contribution to the proportional odds models of the conventional measures of class and employment status and our new measures. Predictably, long-term health status had a powerful independent relationship to report of recent illness in both women and men, in all the models. However, controlling for this effect, all the new measures made a significant additional contribution to the model amongst women. Indeed, both the physical conditions of formal labour and domestic labour conditions were associated with a greater increase in risk than long-term health status. In contrast, amongst men, the new measures did not perform so well. Only domestic conditions made an independent contribution to the model which was approaching significance. Amongst both women and men, the traditional measures of formal working conditions – class and employment status – failed to make a significant independent contribution to the models.

In terms of the relative risks associated with different dimensions of labour conditions, our work suggests that for women the physical conditions of formal labour are associated with the greatest increase in relative risk, followed by domestic labour conditions, whilst the psychosocial conditions of formal labour was associated with the smallest increase. The pattern for men is slightly different. Finally, in our analysis, we found no evidence of an interaction between domestic labour conditions and conditions of labour in paid employment.

In considering these results we would stress our serious reservations about the short-term health state measure available in LSLS. As we have already noted, a measure of recent restricting illness will be confounded with illness behaviour and therefore with the occupancy of different social roles. Though it might be expected that this would be less of a problem with our new measures than with traditional measures, notably employment status, it would have been preferable to have had access to an alternative health state measure, such as a symptom checklist. This would also have allowed us to look separately at different dimensions of ill health – the physical and the psychosocial – which our work on other data sets suggests is important.

That said we would suggest that our findings are of considerable interest to those concerned with better understanding the social patterning of health and illness between women and men and between different social classes. The advantage of developing a unified measure of labour demands and conditions was never intended to be technical, but rather to be of theoretical substance: such measures allow a direct comparison of women's and men's health. This paper and the analysis it presented has shown that there are many problems to be overcome in this endeavour, including developing better measures of ill-health. But it is clear that the labour conditions measures result in a superior model to that derived using conventional measures for women, and in men they perform no worse. These findings indicate that the theoretical advantages of the approach developed here can be safely pursued – albeit perhaps best done so via the collection of new data.

Acknowledgements

This research was undertaken as part of an ESRC funded research project at the Thomas Coram Research Unit under grant number R000231774. We are grateful to Peter Townsend for permission to use the London Standard of Living Survey, to Ian Plewis of the Thomas Coram Research Unit, London, and to Alan Rigby of ARC Research Unit, Manchester, for statistical advice.

References

Arber, S., Gilbert, N. and Dale, A. (1985), 'Paid employment and women's health: a benefit or a source of role strain?', *Sociology of Health and Illness*, **7**:375.

Bartley, M., Popay, J. and Plewis, I. (1992), 'Domestic conditions, paid employment and women's experience of ill-health', *Sociology of Health and Illness*, **14**, (3).

Bartley, M. and Owen, C. (1991), 'Selection and privilege: the relationship between health, occupation and economic activity', unpublished paper, Thomas Coram Research Unit, University of London.

Baruch, G.K., Biener, L. and Barnett, R.C. (1987), 'Women and gender in research and work and family stress', *American Psychologist*, **42**, (2): 130–136.
Blaxter, M. (1990), *Health and Lifestyles*, London: Routledge.
Bottomore, T. and Rubel, M. (1963), *Karl Marx: Selected Writings in Sociology and Social Philosophy*, Harmondsworth: Pelican.
Boulton, M. (1986), *On becoming a mother*, London: Tavistock.
Brown, G. and Harries, T. (1979), *Social origins of depression: a study of psychiatric disorder in women*, London: Tavistock.
Celantano, D.D., Linet, M.S. and Stewart, W.F. (1990), 'Gender differences in the experience of headache', *Social Science and Medicine*, **12**:1289–1295.
Cooper, C.L. and Smith, M.J. (1985), *Job Stress and Blue Collar Work*, London: Wiley.
Davey-Smith, G., Bartley, M. and Blane, D. (1990), 'The Black Report on inequalities in health: 10 years on', *British Medical Journal*, 373–377.
Dex, S. (1985), *The Sexual Division of Work*, Harvester Press.
Finch, J. and Groves, D. (eds) (1983), *A Labour of Love; Women, Work and Caring*, London: Routledge and Kegan Paul.
Fox, J. and Goldblatt, P. (1982), *Longitudinal Study: Socio-demographic mortality differentials 1971–75 England and Wales*, London: HMSO.
Gove, W. and Hughes, M. (1981), 'Beliefs versus data: more on the illness behaviour of men and women', *American Sociological Review*, **46**:123–8.
Graham, H. (1983), 'Caring: a labour of love', in Finch, J. and Groves, D. (eds), *A Labour of Love; Women, Work and Caring*, London: Routledge and Kegan Paul.
Graham, H. (1985), *Caring for the family*, Health Education Council Research Monograph 1.
Hall, E.M. (1989), 'Gender, work control and stress: a theoretical discussion and an empirical test', *International Journal of Health Services*, **19**, (4): 725–745.
Karasek, R.A. (1979), 'Job demands, job decision latitude and mental strain: implications for job re-design', *Administrative Science Quarterly*, **24**:285–308.
Karasek, R.A. (1989), 'The political implications of psychosocial work and redesign: a model of the psychosocial class structure', *International Journal of Health Services*, **19**, (3):481–508.
Karasek, R.A., Baker, K., Maxer, F., Ahlbom, A. and Theorell, T. (1981), 'Job-decision, job demands and cardiovascular disease: a propective study of Swedish men', *American Journal of Public Health*, **71**:694–705.
Karasek, R.A. *et al.* (1983), 'Patterns of health associated with work and family stressors for male and female Swedish white collar workers', New York: Columbia University, Department of Industrial Engineering and Operations Research.
Koskenvuo, M., Kaprio, J., Lonnquist, J. and Sarna, S. (1986), 'Social factors and the gender difference in mortality', *Social Science and Medicine*, **23**, (6):605–609.
Kowarzik, U. and Popay, J. (1989), *'That's women's work': report on women's unpaid labour in the home*, Employment and Training Group, London Resource Centre.
Marmot, M. (1987), 'Look after your heart: stress and cardiovascular disease – a studiable case?', *Health Trends*, **19**:21–25.

Marmot, M., Shipley, M.J. and Rose, G. (1984), 'Inequalities in health – specific explanations or a general pattern?', *Lancet*, **1**:1003–6.
Martin, C.J., Platt, S.D. and Hunt, S.M. (1987), 'Housing conditions and ill-health', *British Medical Journal*, **294**:1125–7.
Oakley, A. (1974), *Housework*, Harmondsworth: Penguin.
Owen, J. (1987), *Survey of Living Standards in London: Fieldwork Report*, London Research Centre/London Residuary Body.
Popay, J. and Bartley, M. (1989), 'Conditions of labour and women's health', in Martin, C. and McQueen, D. (eds), *Readings for a New Public Health*, Edinburgh: Edinburgh University Press, pp. 89–97.
Popay, J., Bartley, M. and Owen, C. (1993), 'Gender inequalities in health: social position, affective disorders and minor physical morbidity', *Social Science and Medicine*, **36**, (1): 21–32.
Roberts, H. (1987), 'Women and social classification', in Keil, T. and Bytheway, B. (eds), *Sociology of Lifestyle*, Basingstoke: Macmillan.
Roberts, H. (1990), *Women's Health Counts*, London: Heinemann.
Rosenfeld, S. (1989), 'The effects of women's employment: personal control and sex differences in mental health', *Journal of Health and Social Behaviour*, **30**:77–91.
Silman, A. (1987), 'Why do women live longer and is it worth it?', *British Medical Journal*, **294**:1311–1312.
Spring-Rice Davies, M. (1939), *Working Class Wives*, Harmondsworth: Penguin.
Townsend, P. (1979), *Poverty in the United Kingdom*, Harmondsworth: Penguin.
Townsend, P. (1990), *Deprivation and Ill-health: New Scientific Evidence and Implications for Policy*, Institute for Health Policy Studies, Occasional Paper.
Verbrugge, L.M. (1983), 'Multiple roles and the health of women', *Journal of Health and Social Behaviour*, **24**:16–30.
Verbrugge, L.M. (1987), 'Role responsibilities, role burdens and physical health', in Crosby, F.J. (ed.), *Spouse, Parent, Worker*, London/Yale: Yale University Press.
Verbrugge, L.M. (1989), 'The twain meet: empirical explanations of sex differences in health and mortality', *Journal of Health and Social Behaviour*, **30**:283–304.
Whitehead, M. (1987), *The Health Divide: Inequalities in Health in the 1980s*, London: Health Education Council.
Wilkinson, R. (1986), 'Income and Mortality', in Wilkinson, R. (ed.), *Class and Health: Research and Longitudinal Data*, London: Tavistock.
Wilkinson, R. (1990), *Income and Mortality: A Natural Experiment*, Centre for Medical Research, University of Sussex.

7 Health issues in male early retirement

Dallas Cliff

Introduction

It is now increasingly unlikely that adult males will continue working in one lifetime occupational career to the statutory age of retirement at 65. Up until the 1980s, a breakdown in health was the major factor in early withdrawal from the labour market, but this is less often so nowadays, given the proliferation of national and company-based early retirement schemes during the last decade.

An older literature suggested that until the 1980s, early retirement was almost always connected to a breakdown in health. Steiner and Dorfman (1957) found that 79 per cent of early retirements were the result of some kind of breakdown in health whilst Shanas *et al.* (1968) found that 61 per cent of early retirements in Denmark were health-related, as opposed to 50 per cent in the United States and 44 per cent in the United Kingdom. Parker (1982) found that ill health continued to be a major factor in early retirement in the United Kingdom during the late 1970s.

More recent research has added the consideration of personal financial security to that of health, as the prime factors in early retirement decisions. In the United States, a lively exchange has taken place between Kingson (1981, 1982a, 1982b, 1983) and Myers (1982, 1983). Kingson argued that poor health was the overriding consideration whilst Myers maintained that economic factors were most salient, as individuals reacted to national and corporate incentives. Kingson's case rested on survey studies of early retirees and on subsequent mortality data. Myers maintained that health complaints were often used as post-decisional rationalizations, and argued that mortality statistics did not show significant differences between early retirees and other groups. His strongest argument, however, was that the rising tide of early retirement could hardly be explained by a deterioration in health standards. Subsequent research has tended to support Myers. Daymont and Andrisani (1983) did not find early retirees markedly less healthy than those who continued working, a finding supported by research based on cohort comparisons (Baker *et al.* 1982). Bazzoli (1985), using more sensitive health indicators than crude mortality statistics concluded with Myers that health was a less significant factor than financial provision.

Philipson (1990) has claimed in the context of the United Kingdom that those taking early retirement as a result of favourable financial incentives are in the minority, in relation to 'a much larger number who retire early because of health problems' (p. 152). This seems unlikely, as will be seen, for it would require that the decreasing participation rate of older workers be understood in terms of a widespread deterioration in health. More recently Laczko and Phillipson (1991) have reported Labour Force Survey data on early exit from the work force, suggesting that for men in the 60–64 age range 9 per cent of non-manual and 19 per cent of manual workers gave ill-health as the main reason for leaving their last job (p. 74). However, it may well be the case that increasing financial provision for early retirement may enable men to respond to their health needs by giving up work, an option that may have been unavailable in previous decades.

This chapter explores the continuing importance of health issues in early retirement through an analysis of three recent studies. Firstly, McGoldrick and Cooper's (1988) ESRC funded survey based on 120 pilot interviews and the distribution of questionnaires to 1,800 early retired men drawn from 17 different companies known to be operating early retirement schemes. Secondly, private research undertaken by the author on behalf of a major motor manufacturer, involved 30 pilot interviews and a survey of 300 employees during the months of them actually taking early retirement in 1988, and 30 pilot interviews and a survey of 2,000 employees who had taken early retirement from the company between 1982 and 1987. Thirdly, the author's doctoral research (Cliff 1989) involved the analysis of 50 depth interviews with men who had taken early retirement from a chemical plant in West Yorkshire between 1980 and 1986. These will be referred to as the ESRC study, the Motor Industry study and the West Yorkshire study, respectively. It should be noted that health issues were not the major focus in any of these studies, but they all included the consideration of health issues as a subsidiary theme. To that extent, they might usefully provide the basis for a tentative and exploratory analysis of health issues, in relation to male early retirement.

One important effect of contemporary social and economic change has been to call into question the notion that lifelong paid employment will constitute the typical work career of most men (Tolson 1977). Some commentators have suggested that such changes lie behind the current problematization of notions of masculinity (Hearn 1987). The focus in this chapter on male early retirement is not intended to suggest that early retirement is not an issue for older female workers, but rather that the problems faced by men and women are different and that the gendered nature of contemporary society demands that, initially, a separate analysis be undertaken.

The chapter will argue on the basis of evidence from these three studies that early retirement differs from conventional retirement, in that early retirees are generally healthier, more affluent and active in terms of both leisure and further paid employment, but that older patterns of health-related early retirement still persist for a significant minority, and that this relates closely to social class background with manual workers being far more likely to replicate these earlier patterns. It will draw on the concept of 'career' (Becker 1963; Abrams 1982) as a fruitful means of linking the way individuals negotiate their changed circumstances with the wider social factors that structure those transitions for particular age groups, generations and social classes.

It will argue that, whilst most early retirees go on to negotiate varied careers which mix family and leisure pursuits, short-term and part-time employment and voluntary work in ways that are generally highly satisfying, others, mainly manual workers, experience early retirement in terms of ill health careers that cut down their options and leave them financially and socially impoverished. The chapter supports Philipson's (1990) contention that there is a widening divide between those middle-aged retirees 'who will develop a leisure-orientated lifestyle, built around the expanding consumer market aimed at the over-50s' (p. 159) and those who are reproducing earlier patterns of health-related early retirement.

However, the evidence from these three studies also suggests that one aspect of the careers of some middle-aged male early retirees is that, faced with problems of sickness and ill health in their own families, they see themselves as available in the role of carers in ways that similar men in full-time employment do not. If changes in patterns of employment are restructuring gender divisions in contemporary society and undermining the notion of paid work as the lifelong career of the 'breadwinner male', then the experience of these men becomes highly salient in any discussion of the ways in which these changes are being worked out by people in their everyday lives.

The background to the growth of early retirement

The last decade has seen a substantial reduction in the economic participation rates of older workers. Much, though not all of this reduction has been due to the widespread use of early retirement but, with some notable exceptions (Atkinson 1985; Laczko and Walker 1985; McGoldrick and Cooper 1980, 1988; Parker 1982; Walker 1982, 1985; Wood 1980) it has not been widely discussed in social scientific literature. As Table 1 shows, the rate for men over the age of sixty has fallen from 80.4 per cent in 1976 to 55.0 per cent in 1988.

Table 1 Civilian labour force economic activity rates for males over forty-five, selected years 1976–88, projections for 1991 and 2000 (percentages)

Year	Males 45–59 years	Males 60–65 years	Males 65+
1976	94.9	80.4	14.5
1981	93.0	69.3	10.3
1984	90.9	59.4	8.1
1988	87.8	55.0	8.0
Projections			
1991	88.4	55.0	6.8
2000	87.7	53.9	4.4

Source: Social Trends (1990) CSO, 70.

The British experience is consistent with trends in both Europe (Cribier 1981; Blyton 1983; Laczko and Walker 1985; Olson-Frick 1980, 1985) and the United States (Kestenbaum 1985; Myers 1982). In both the United States and Sweden, early retirement policies have been pursued in the context of age discrimination legislation, but Sweden seems to be alone in promoting 'flexible retirement' through a scheme enabling older workers to draw a partial pension whilst working a 17 hour week (Laczko and Walker 1985).

National government in Britain has encouraged early retirement as a way of creating jobs for younger workers but this has often been in conflict with the policies of individual companies, who have seen early retirement as a means of cutting down the overall size of the work force (Blyton 1983). It is an expensive policy pursued mainly in the public sector and by larger companies and has been aimed largely, although not exclusively, at salaried managerial and professional workers (Atkinson 1985; Walker 1975). Despite its cost, early retirement has been an attractive policy for companies, in that it enables 'headcount reduction' to take place without undue opposition from work forces and Trade Unions. More recently, early retirement has spread to wider groups of workers (McGoldrick and Cooper 1988), although manual workers are likely to be offered less attractive schemes (Atkinson 1985). Most schemes are voluntary: personnel managers talk of 'opening the early retirement window' to describe schemes where financial incentives, such as enhanced pensions and generous 'golden handshakes', are offered until a predesignated target number of retirements has been achieved. Once this has occurred, the 'window' is closed. If insufficient people come forward the window can be opened further by increasing the incentives (Gravitz and Rumack 1983).

Health in relation to the early retirement decision

The three studies that form the basis of the discussion here suggest a decreased, but still significant, role of health breakdown in the early retirement decision. The ESRC study found that ill health prior to retirement was a consideration for 23.7 per cent of respondents and a major factor for 15.7 per cent. This factor was found to be associated with the growth of problems in coping with the job which increased the motivation to seek early retirement. The salience of health concerns was strongly associated with lower social class groups ($p = .001$) whilst higher social class groups were more highly associated with the decisional factor 'own finances right' ($p = .001$). However, it should be noted that the proportion of respondents reporting a breakdown in health as the major factor in the decision is substantially less than in the earlier studies cited above.

A similar pattern emerged from the Motor Industry study where ill health was reported as being a very important factor in the decision by 19.3 per cent of respondents and the most important factor by 13 per cent. Again this was related to social class with 16.9 per cent of manual respondents and 5.5 per cent of non-manual respondents claiming this as the most important factor ($p = .0365$). This study found that those for whom ill health was the major factor were also taking early retirements in circumstances which they saw as far less well resourced. Only 12 per cent of those from whom ill health was not a factor rated their financial package as 'not at all adequate' whilst this was true of 33.3 per cent of those for whom ill health was a major factor. As Table 2 illustrates, these men were also likely to be taking early retirement because work was becoming too demanding, the job had changed for the worse or because they feared for their future health.

The West Yorkshire study also found ill health to be a more salient factor for male manual workers. Whilst 25 per cent of these men from the chemical industry reported ill health as a major factor in the decision, as Table 3 shows, there was a highly significant difference between manual and salaried men.

For the men for whom ill health was the major factor in the decision, there was no sense that they were taking an active decision. As one man put it.

Table 2 **Factors in the early retirement decision related to having ill health as an important factor (percentages of those rating each factor as important)**

The Motor Industry Study

	Ill health not a major factor	**Ill health a major factor**
Other factors also rated as important		
Work too demanding	20.83%	58.33%
Job changed for worse	17.6%	35.19%
Fear for future health	8.4%	81.48%
(N=285)		

Table 3 **The relationship between occupational status and having a breakdown in health as the major factor in the early retirement decision (numbers of men)**

The West Yorkshire Study

	Occupational status	
	Non-manual	**Manual**
Health the major factor	1	9
Health not the major factor	19	11
Total	20	20

Note: Chi-square = 6.533 DF:1 p = .0106 with continuity correction.

> I didn't retire voluntary. My health gave me no option. I might have taken early retirement eventually but at least I'd have been able to pick my own time. (Manual – skilled)

Others were well aware that in previous decades men like themselves had been routinely given light duties on the plant and bitterly recognized that 'times had changed'.

> I didn't want to finish. I thought I'd just get put on light duties but I was told that just wasn't possible in the present financial climate. (Manual – skilled)

> The works doctor diagnosed me and I was told I'd have to go. At one time they'd have made you a gardener or something but not now. (Manual – skilled)

These differences in the salience of health for the two groups are highly significant and reinforce the general picture of class and occupational differences in health reported by the Black Report and the Health Divide (Wilkinson 1986; Townsend *et al.* (1988). These reports have given rise to a number of debates, as to whether these differences should be explained and understood in terms of material factors such as working conditions, or as the outcome of differences in diet and lifestyle. These debates cannot be resolved by using the data from this relatively small study, but a number of observations can be made. It was certainly the opinion of these men that their health problems were the result of the physically arduous nature of their work and exposure to hazardous chemicals rather than to 'unhealthy' or 'irresponsible' lifestyles away from work. In two cases, men with breathing problems had proved a link with the escape of poisonous fumes in areas in which they were working and had received extra compensation as a result. The others displayed a mixture of heart disease, strokes, back and muscular problems associated with heavy physical work.

Several men, four manual and one non-manual, reported that their early retirement decision was health related in the prophylactic sense in that, although they felt healthy, they feared that if they did not take early retirement they might not retire in good health. This was often related to fears concerning parents and relatives who had 'died in harness'.

> My father died the day his first pension arrived. I always intended to take early retirement as soon as possible. (Non-manual – foreman)

> My father and two uncles died early having worked all their lives and I thought I'm not going to have that. As soon as I can get a golden handshake I'm off. (Non-manual – manager)

On the whole, the Motor Industry study and the West Yorkshire study suggest a marked difference between proactive non-manual men for whom early retirement is the outcome of a long-term personal and financial plan and the more reactive manual men for whom early retirement arises out of immediate circumstances of which ill health remains an important factor. Perhaps the most poignant illustration of these differences is illustrated by the fact that those who retired through ill health were far less likely to see early retirement as an occasion for celebration ($p = .0113$). As one man in this position said:

> Celebrate? You must be joking! I didn't feel as if I had anything to celebrate about. (Hourly – skilled)

A further health factor in the early retirement decision revealed in the ESRC and Motor Industry studies, was the ill health of wives where the primary motivation to take early retirement was so that the man was able to care for his sick wife. In the ESRC study this was a major factor in 10.3 per cent of cases, whilst in the Motor Industry study it was reported as the most important factor by 9.3 per cent of the men. In the latter study there was a significant social class difference with 14.5 per cent of manual men as against only 2.6 per cent of non-manual men reporting this as a major factor ($p = .0066$). Although, clearly a less significant factor than the men's own health, it nonetheless represents a significant minority and highlights the role of some early retired men as carers within the family. I will return to this theme later in this chapter.

Ill health and satisfaction with early retirement

The foregoing section suggests a significant difference between those men for whom early retirement is a positive decision based on attractive financial incentives and those for whom the decision is forced through ill health. Not surprisingly, this dichotomy in experience continues through into the experience of early retirement and is a major factor in explaining levels of satisfaction and dissatisfaction. Experience in early retirement seems to reflect the more general polarization of contemporary British society, noted by a number of commentators (Pahl 1984).

The ESRC study found levels of satisfaction with early retirement to be generally high, with 80 per cent of their sample reporting themselves to be 'definitely satisfied'. Satisfaction revolved around factors such as having more freedom and leisure time, being able to spend more time with one's family and having more social contact. In attempting to unravel the main factors related to dissatisfaction, McGoldrick and Cooper identified ill health as one of the three most important factors, along with 'money worries' and feeling bored and depressed. These factors will clearly be interrelated, as ill health typically forces early retirement on grounds other than attractive financial incentives and leaves retirees short of both material resources and physical energy.

The Motor Industry study also revealed relatively high levels of satisfaction with 35 per cent reporting themselves very satisfied and a further 45 per cent quite satisfied. The factors which gave rise to general satisfaction were similar to the ESRC study with free time, the ability to persue non-work interests and time to spend with family and friends predominating. Again, however, those for whom early retirement was based on ill health were far more likely to be dissatisfied. Of those for whom ill health was a major factor in the decision, 35 per cent reported themselves highly satisfied with the decision overall, as opposed to 58 per cent of those for whom this was not the case ($p = .0001$). This could be explained, to a very great extent, by the inferior financial position of those who had retired through ill health. Only 56 per cent of those with ill health as the major factor reported feeling satisfied with their level of financial security, as opposed to 79 per cent of those for whom it was not a factor. This financial insecurity was reflected in the different ways in which lump sum payments were used. Those retiring through ill health were less likely to invest this money and were more likely to use it to pay off existing commitments.

Those who had retired through ill health further reported themselves to be less satisfied with the way they spent their time ($p = .0001$), less satisfied with the way they got on with their families ($p = .0109$), less satisfied with the contact they had with ex-workmates ($p = .0082$) and had more problems with tax and social security ($p = .0149$).

The Motor Industry study, in common with the ESRC study, found that many early retirees returned to paid employment and that the ability to find part-time or short-term contract work was also closely related to levels of satisfaction. This finding was reinforced in the West Yorkshire study on the basis of which it was suggested that one important pattern in early retirement careers was for healthy men with marketable skills to negotiate their own 'flexible' retirements. Such men would typically have high levels of involvement in paid employment in the early years of their retirement and withdraw at their own pace by, for instance, increasing the time between short-term contracts. Such flexible strategies are obviously not open to those for whom ill health precludes further paid work.

The West Yorkshire study attempted to go beyond the simple reporting of satisfaction by questionnaire response, by using qualitative data collected in depth interviews to construct a 'quality of life index' based on the overall pattern of the respondent's assessment of his situation (Cliff 1989). On this basis, four broad categories of experience were identified: Category A, where quality of life was highly acceptable, in which respondents perceived early retirement very positively and held few if any negative views; Category B, where quality of life was acceptable, in which respondents expressed themselves very positively whilst acknowledging some negative feelings about loss of income, social status and isolation; Category C, where quality of life was merely tolerable, in which respondents were more concerned with loss of income, status, absence of social contacts and problems with family relationships, and who felt themselves to be very much 'making the best of things'; Category D, where quality of life was very poor, in which respondents expressed serious misgivings about early retirement and viewed the whole experience very negatively. Where they had taken early retirement through choice, they saw themselves as having made a very great mistake; where they had taken it because of ill health, they saw themselves as very unfortunate. The relationship between these categories of experience and the importance of health to the retirement decision with 87 per cent of those for whom ill health was not a major factor in the top two categories as opposed to only 30 per cent of those for whom ill health was a major factor in the decision.

Financial problems predominated in the accounts of the men with ill health problems. One man who had suffered a heart attack had been advised by his doctor to take up golf as a form of exercise. But things did not work out for him:

> I love sport. I took up golf and went to lessons but when I finished I realized that I just couldn't afford to set myself up, to join a club and get a decent set of clubs. (Manual – skilled)

For this man, financial retrenchment led to a more privatized existence. He and his wife explained that they 'just made ends meet' but at the cost of 'getting out and doing things'.

> We have less money now. We look after the pennies and that curtails your enjoyment. Trips off to York and the races are off now. The money wasn't quite enough to fill the gap.

Another man who had also suffered from a heart attack faced similar problems:

> A pension isn't the same as a full wage. I've still got some (lump sum) money put away but not enough. It wasn't until I finished physiotherapy that it hit home and then the bottom of the world fell out. (Manual – skilled)

In his case too, financial restrictions led to social isolation:

> We can't afford to mix socially very often. I rarely see people. The dog's my only outlet now: I go further and further with him.

The stress of these problems effected other family members. The wife of another man who had retired through ill health confided:

> I've been sick with worry. I've been off work with a nervous breakdown. We had such a lot of words. That money was all we had. I've got to give up work soon and I just don't know how we'll manage then. (Wife/manual – skilled)

Health restrictions also gave rise to feelings of not being able to participate fully in a satisfactory mix of activities. The following man did not feel financially deprived, but his health was poor and his mobility restricted. A bachelor living alone, his daily routine was tolerable but he described it overall as 'surviving, not really living any more'. He had developed a mode of life that almost completely reversed day and night.

> All the days are the same. I go to bed at 7 am and get up at 3 pm. I have All-Bran and a cup of water and a bacon sandwich for breakfast. Then I potter about. I have to keep moving so I catch the bus to the local baths at 6.30 and have a gentle swim. And then I'm back at 7.30 and in the pub across the road. I drink four or five pints of beer, smoke three or four cigars and play pool. When the pub closes I come back home and watch the video of the night's television. I usually just leave it on Channel 4. I like the documentaries, the nature programmes, the historical things and the politics. (Manual – unskilled)

Thus, ill health is no longer the major reason for taking early retirement for the majority of men, it remains the case that for those men who do retire for this reason their quality of life is likely to be low through a combination of factors. Ill health often forces early retirement on financial terms which would not normally be considered viable: it precludes those periods of intermittent paid employment often used by early retirees to 'top up' their pensions: this lack of financial resources, coupled with a lack of vitality and mobility often leads to social isolation. The comparison of their condition with that of healthy, affluent, leisured early retirees only makes their plight harder to bear.

Health in early retirement

For the fortunate majority for whom early retirement is a largely positive experience, increased physical well being and better health is an important benefit. In the ESRC study over half reported better health since retirement, with 25.4 per cent seeing it as a major benefit. Specific health benefits reported were: better appetite, sleeping better, being able to take more exercise, feeling less tired, experiencing less stress and having fewer worries. The Motor Industry study included no direct questions on changes in health status, but the West Yorkshire study reinforced this picture.

Most of the men in this study felt that they had become less tense and irritable, more relaxed and easier to live with. This theme emerged in the interviews of all 29 cases that were assigned to the two highest quality of life categories.

> I feel less pressured. I have a greater sense of well being. I feel more relaxed. (Non-manual – technical)

> I feel more calm and relaxed. When I was working I used to bring work home with me. I used to think about it all night. That's all gone. I'm more even tempered but perhaps that's old age. (Manual – semi-skilled)

> I'm older, lazier, more relaxed but I doubt if I've changed in other ways. (Non-manual – manager)

One wife endorsed this view with regard to her husband:

> He would come home and relive the day in his mind and not talk to me. He's a lot easier to live with now. (Manual – unskilled)

One manager commented on the absence of the 'Sunday night feeling':

> On Sunday night the tension grew. I became different mentally – geared up for Monday morning. Now Sunday evening is as enjoyable as any other. (Non-manual – manager)

A substantial number of men said that they felt healthier as a result of taking early retirement. Only seven reported a worsening of health, whilst 16 reported that it had improved, and another 16 that it had stayed the same. There was no relationship between present reported health and having ill health as a major factor in the early retirement decision, although none of those who retired on health grounds actually reported worsening health. The men who did report worsening health were all previously healthy and had contracted some specific complaint such as ulcers, back and heart problems since retirement.

The general pattern that emerges, then, is one of the majority of early retired men reporting health benefits in early retirement, based on a release from the stresses and tensions associated with their occupational roles. The generally high levels of satisfaction with early retirement revealed by these studies is clearly based on the fact that most have experienced an increase in feelings of health, vitality and well-being. Indeed, the success of the enterprise is largely measured in those terms. A successful early retirement is almost, by definition, a healthy early retirement. This majority experience stands in stark contradistinction to that of that minority for whom the central feature of early retirement was the adjustment to and reconciliation with a breakdown in health.

Early retired men as carers

The conventional sociological wisdom that most informal care within households is provided by women (Briggs 1983; Ungerson 1987) has been challenged by Arber and Gilbert on the basis of evidence provided by the General Household Survey (1989a, 1989b). They suggest that at least a third of carers of the infirm elderly are male and that male spouses are as likely to be caring for an infirm partner as the reverse. Nor are male carers likely to receive more support from social services when the severity of illness is taken into account. They do, however, suggest that the reasons for becoming a carer may differ along the gender dimension, with men taking over a caring role in the context of a long-term relationship in which ill health results in a relationship of mutual support becoming one of dependency. Women, on the other hand, are more likely to become carers out of a sense of social obligation with elderly dependents entering households to receive care. In short, men become carers out of love, whilst women become carers through duty.

The data from these three studies support the view that older men are likely to be involved in giving care. The analysis of the early retirement decision revealed that a small, but significant, proportion of men gave the need to look after a sick wife as one of their major reasons for taking early retirement. Both the ESRC study and the Motor Industry study found that spending more time with, and supporting, one's family were perceived as important positive advantages of taking early retirement. The West Yorkshire study provided the opportunity to gather more qualitative data on the involvement of the sample in care within their families.

Altogether 32 per cent of the sample (14 men) had been involved in providing care. Four were involved in the full-time care of invalid wives and one further man had done so until his wife's death. A further four men reported periods when they had taken over the role of houseworker and carer during their wives' illnesses. Finally, five men *had* looked after, or *were* looking after, relatives outside their immediate nuclear families. In four cases, this was their own mother or mother-in-law and, in one case, an aunt. The freedom to give such care without a great deal of disruption was one of the most positive aspects of early retirement.

> It (early retirement DC) was a godsend when my mother got ill. I visited her every day for two years. Lord knows how we would have managed if I'd still been working. (Non-manual – manager)

> I've got a mother who is just going through the stage of not coping very well. We've just got her into a place and we've been clearing the house. That's taken a lot of evenings. I've been on that every evening of last week. I don't know how I'd have coped if I'd been working. (Non-manual – manager)

All the men who had wives with permanent ill health had taken over the main houseworker role:

> I do all the housework now the wife's ill. I cook, clean, keep it tidy. She's in a wheelchair now so she can do very little herself. She never wanted me to do it when she was ill. (Manual – semi-skilled)

> My wife is not too well now so I do all the housework. I get up early and see to it and then I'm clear for the day. I do all the washing, cooking, cleaning, vacuuming and all. I never did any of that before apart from washing the odd pot. (Non-manual – manager)

In the case of men who had looked after their wives through periods of illness, they had all reverted to a more traditional masculine role after the illness was over.

> I did everything for three months when she was ill, but as soon as she was better she was back to it. She accused me of trying to push her nose out. (Non-manual – foreman)

For these men, caring for the sick, along with taking the primary responsibility for household and domestic tasks was definitely regarded as 'female' work. In the absence of their own traditional masculine role as 'worker', however, it represented an arena that they were prepared to enter if necessary. Such activity was seen as depending entirely on their having taken early retirement, although the creation of space in which this activity could be taken up was seen as a major benefit of having taken retirement. 'I don't know how I'd have coped if I'd been working' was a major theme for these men.

Conclusion

This chapter has reviewed some of the evidence from three recent studies concerning health issues, in relation to the experience of those men taking early retirement over the last decade. The earlier pattern of a breakdown in health being the major reason for the majority of early retirements seems to have been replaced by one in which early retirement has been more typically taken on the basis of financial incentives and the desire for leisure or at least some measure of disengagement from a full-time involvement in paid employment. Such men have typically evolved early retirement careers that revolve around leisure, relaxation, free time, and family centredness. The older pattern of financially insecure early retirements, based on a breakdown in health, continues, however, to be an important aspect of the experience of a significant minority of working class men, and reinforces the view that the manual/non-manual divide is of continuing significance to the analysis of inequality in contemporary Britain. Such men are likely to experience much lower levels of satisfaction and quality of life in early retirement. For them, adjustment to ill health and associated deprivation is the central feature of their retirement careers.

For the more fortunate majority, early retirement is associated with a reduction in levels of tension and stress and an improvement in health. The increased importance of the family means that some of these men are themselves involved in a certain amount of care in their own families, mainly in relation to ill and dependent wives, but also in relation to older relatives, particularly their own mothers. Whilst such work is still regarded as traditionally 'female', they do perceive themselves as available for such work in a way that would clearly have been inconceivable if they were still committed to their own full-time occupational roles, and it is clear that these men were by no means without a sense of 'duty' to their wider families. If the 'new man' is anything more than a figment of the media and advertising industries, then he is perhaps more likely to be a retired 52 year old rather than a younger man. As one respondent from the West Yorkshire study so succinctly expressed himself:

> There's one good thing – more than anything I've become aware of families and human things. (Non-manual – manager)

Acknowledgements

I would like to thank Graham Gibbs and Geoff Sparks for their comments on an earlier draft of this paper.

References

Abrams, P. (1982), *Historical Sociology*, Shepton Mallet: Open Books.

Arber, S. and Gilbert, N. (1989a), 'Men: the forgotten carers', *Sociology*, **23**:111–119.

Arber, S. and Gilbert, N. (1989b), 'Transitions in caring: gender, life course and the care of the elderly', in Bytheway, B., Keil, T., Allatt, P. and Bryman, A., *Becoming and Being Old: Sociological Approaches to Later Life*, London: Sage.

Atkinson, J. (1985), *Early Retirement*, IMS Report No. 94, Falmer: Institute of Manpower Studies, University of Sussex.

Baker, D., Packard, M., Radar, A., Reno, U. and Upp, M. (1982), 'Mortality and early retirement', *Social Security Bulletin*, **45**:3–10.

Bazzoli, G. (1985), 'The early retirement decision: new empirical evidence on the influence of health', *Journal of Human Resources*, **20**:214–234.

Becker, H. (1963), *Outsiders: Studies in the Sociology of Deviance*, New York: Free Press.

Blyton, P. (1983), 'Early retirement: an EEC perspective', *The Three Banks Review*, **136**:32–44.

Briggs, A. (1983), *Who Cares?*, Chatham, Kent: Association of Carers.

Cliff, D.R. (1989), 'Life after work: an investigation of men in early retirement', unpublished Ph.D. thesis CNAA: Polytechnic of Huddersfield/University of Manchester.

Cribier, F. (1981), 'Changing retirement patterns in the seventies: the example of a generation of Parisian salaried workers', *Ageing and Society*, **1**:51–72.

Daymont, T. and Andrisani, P. (1983), 'The health and economic status of very early retirees', *Ageing and Work*, **6**:117–135.

Gravitz, D.H. and Rumack, F.W. (1983), 'Opening the early retirement window', *Personnel*, **60**:53–57.

Hearn, J. (1987), *The Gender of Oppression: Men, Masculinity and the Critique of Marxism*, Brighton: Wheatsheaf.

Kestenbaum, B. (1985), 'The measurement of early retirement', *Journal of the American Statistical Society*, **80**:38–45.

Kingson, E.R. (1981), 'Retirement circumstances of very early retirees: A life cycle perspective', *Ageing and Work*, **4**:161–74.

Kingson, E.R. (1982a), 'The health of very early retirees', *Social Security Bulletin*, **54**:3–9.

Kingson, E.R. (1982b), 'Health and the early retirement decision, 1 – critique of early retirement study disputed', *Ageing and Work*, **5**:93–110.

Kingson, E.R. (1983), 'Still more on early retirement', *Ageing and Work*, **6** (2): 111–5.

Laczko, F. and Phillipson, P. (1991), *Changing Work and Retirement*, Milton Keynes: Open University Press.

Laczko, F. and Walker, A. (1985), 'Excluding older workers from the labour market: early retirement in Britain, France and Sweden', in Jones, C. and Brenton, M. (eds), *The Year Book of Social Policy in Britain*, London: Routledge and Kegan Paul.

McGoldrick, A. and Cooper, C. (1980), 'Voluntary early retirement: taking the decision', *Employment Gazette*, August, 854–59.

McGoldrick, A. and Cooper, C. (1988), *Early Retirement*, Aldershot: Gower.

Myers, R.J. (1982), 'Health and the early retirement decision debate. Why do people retire early from work?', *Ageing and Work*, **5**:39–55.

Myers, R.J. (1983), 'More about the controversy on early retirement', *Ageing and Work*, **5**:105–9.

Olson-Frick, H. (1980), 'Early retirement an international perspective', *International Journal of Rehabilitation Research*, **3**:215–23.

Olson-Frick, H. (1985), 'Early retirement an international perspective 2', *International Journal of Rehabilitation Research*, **8**:161–80.

Pahl, R.E. (1984), *Divisions of Labour*, Oxford: Basil Blackwell.

Parker, S. (1982), *Work and Retirement*, London: George Allen and Unwin.

Philipson, C. (1990), 'The Sociology of Retirement', in Bond, J. and Coleman, P., *Ageing in Society: An Introduction to Social Gerontology*, London: Sage.
Shanas, E., Townsend, P., Wedderburn, D., Friis, H., Milhoj, P. and Stenhouner, J. (1968), *Old People in Three Industrial Societies*, London: Routledge and Kegan Paul.
Steiner, P. and Dorfman, O. (1957), *The Economic Status the Aged*, Berkeley: University of California Press.
Tolson, A. (1977), *The Limits to Masculinity*, London: Tavistock.
Townsend, P., Davidson, N. and Whitehead, M. (1988), *Inequalities in Health: The Black Report and The Health Divide*, Harmondsworth: Penguin.
Ungerson, C. (1987), *Policy is Personal: Sex, Gender and Informal Care*, London: Tavistock.
Walker, A. (1982), 'The social consequences of early retirement', *Political Quarterly*, **53**:61–72.
Walker, A. (1985), 'Early retirement – release or refuge from the labour market', *Quarterly Journal of Social Affairs*, **1**:211–29.
Walker, J.W. (1975), 'New appeal of early retirement', *Business Horizons*, **18**:43–48.
Wilkinson, R.G. (1986), *Class and Health: Research and Longitudinal Data*, London: Tavistock.
Wood, S. (1980), 'Managerial reactions to job redundancy through early retirement', *Sociological Review*, **28**:738–807.

8 Occupational health in the UK gas industry

A study of employer, medical and worker knowledge and action on occupational health in the late nineteenth and early twentieth century

Andrew Watterson

Introduction

This chapter attempts to locate aspects of British occupational health in historical context and explore the processes by which occupational diseases are identified, compensated for and defined. Foucault observed that a disease entity was the product of medical discourse which reflected the dominant mode of thinking in a society. In this context, he specifically looked at the relationship between medicine and the exercise of power in society (Turner 1987:9–17). The social construction of knowledge on occupational health is therefore examined and equally important, so are the mechanisms which lead to 'the social construction of ignorance' (Otway 1985:7).

Research from the United States, Germany, Italy, Australia, France, Canada, Poland and Hungary reveals significant under-reporting of worker action on health and safety (Navarro and Berman 1983; Berman 1978; Gersuny 1981; Nelkin and Brown 1984; Creighton and Gunningham 1985; Nelkin 1985; Bagnara, Misiti and Wintersberger 1985; Judkins 1986; Elling 1986; Rowland 1980). Close attention to the experience of workers, using interviews and other methods, produces valuable studies of workforce problems, attitudes to and actions on occupational health and safety (Nelkin and Brown 1984). Many medical practitioners surprisingly still appear to view this approach as a revolutionary medical method. The exhortations of Bernard Ramazzini in seventeenth century Italy, calling for doctors to ask patients who visited them one question among many – 'What do you do?' – and listen to their replies – seem to have been ignored.

Research findings on worker health and safety action link in with developments in 'popular epidemiology', which has recently been defined as:

> the process by which laypersons gather statistics and other information and also direct and marshal the knowledge and resources of experts in order to understand the epidemiology of disease (Brown 1989:618).

The case study of gas worker action on occupational health presented here is an early example of popular epidemiology which, post-Sellafield and post-Camelford, is springing up in many places to challenge not only traditional epidemiology but also traditional occupational and environmental health. Worker epidemiology has a long history in Western Europe. The Berlin Health Care Association founded by Salomon Neumanns in 1849, and banned four years later, with 9,000 members, because of its 'political' demands for health improvements, involved co-operative medical care between doctors and workers, with workers carrying out their own epidemiological surveys (Labisch 1985:36). The investigations of occupational health issues in Britain by social scientists in an historical context have, however, been limited until recently (Weindling 1985; Watterson 1988). This chapter looks at how occupational health problems were recognized, raised but infrequently solved, by workers and employers in the gas industry.

There have been few studies of health and safety and industrial relations in specific industries: Carson's work on the off-shore oil industry and Codrington and Henley's study of the construction industry are perhaps the most useful. Carson stresses the importance of the Weberian view that 'bureaucracy tends to turn problems of politics into problems of administration' (Carson 1981:9). He looked at how the off-shore oil industry, the legislature, the executive and enforcement agencies dealt with the high fatality and serious injury rate in the industry. The analysis is an important one with reference to the role of the state on health and safety, the close relationship between industry and the government – effectively synonymous, of course, in the gas industry after nationalization – and the 'relative weakness of the organised labour movement'.

Studies on safety representatives in the construction industry after 1974 show the importance of trade union site organization for effective worker involvement on health and safety issues, including problems posed by subcontraction of work, the weaknesses of national union health and safety organization and the problems unions face in maintaining health and safety standards in an economic recession (Codrington and Henley 1981:308).

Recent detailed studies of safety self-regulation since 1974 in the chemicals, construction and retail industries have highlighted the need for more effective health and safety systems at a local level and more national trade union support for trade union safety representatives linked to better information and wider rights – if health and safety at work was to be improved in the UK (Dawson *et al.* 1988:244–281). A study of the chemical industry revealed that no personnel managers questioned about their priorities mentioned either health and safety or working conditions in their lists. First priority was given to labour costs, then strike free production, then low absenteeism and labour turnover (Gill *et al.* 1978:138, 68, 133). This raises doubts about the consultative approach to health and safety based on the Joint Consultative Committee system, joint safety committees which lacked worker confidence and Gill observed that:

> ...identity of interest is a myth, for health and safety considerations are often sacrificed to the demands of production and costs. Health and safety issues demand strong countervailing bargaining powers for employees from union organisation and shop stewards with a willingness to learn and go on learning about safety hazards and hazardous processes (Gill 1978:240).

The Gill analysis confirms earlier work on the chemicals industry (Nichols and Armstrong 1973:6–29) and has much validity for developments in the gas industry too.

Aims and methodology

This study concentrates exclusively on the occupational health problems faced by manual workers in the gas industry, primarily in the General and Municipal Workers Union and does not examine the hazards faced by managerial and office staffs. The key questions raised relate to an attempt to understand the extent to which employers, government, medicine and workers fulfilled Sir Thomas Legge's four axioms of occupational health, particularly the fourth and first axioms. Legge had been the UK's Senior Government Medical Factory Inspector in the early 1920s, and in 1934 in his book 'Industrial Maladies' he noted:

1. Unless and until an employer has done everything – and everything means a good deal – workers can do next to nothing to protect themselves from occupational ill-health although they will be willing to do their share.
2. If influence can be brought to bear on those occupational health factors external to a worker, factors the worker cannot control, occupational hazards can be successfully reduced or removed. If this cannot be done, occupational health policies will never be wholly successful.
3. In cases of dust and fume problems [lead was the case Legge cited], if you stop inhalation, you will stop poisoning.
4. All workers should be told something of the danger of the materials with which they come into contact and not be left to find out for themselves – sometimes at the cost of their lives (Legge 1934:3).

The chapter, therefore, looks at when and why evidence about industrial diseases in the gas industry emerged; how that evidence was gathered and by whom; what obstacles existed to prevent the dissemination of the information; and how the evidence was interpreted, used and by whom.

In 1987, Turner called for sociological eclecticism in the study of diseases. He suggested, for instance, that a sociology of an occupational disease like Repetitive Strain Injury would require:

1 'A phenomenology of pain with a specific inquiry into the sufferer's interpretations and perceptions of the disorder';
2 'an analysis of the social processes by which the 'disease' is constituted as a topic by conflicting professional groups with their own vested interests in the existence or disappearance of the problem';
3 'a political economy of the conditions' ... in modern capitalism which through pressure on the worker, create work processes which produce occupational injuries (Turner 1987:15–16).

The phenomenology of pain is not dealt with here, although the perceptions of gas workers about occupational disease are explored. Turner's other two categories in the context of industrial rather than specifically capitalist society are examined.

Research findings from the Department of Employment's Manuscript books recording industrial disputes, relevant parliamentary papers, medical papers, focused interviews with gas managers at a national level, interviews with and questionnaires from trade union safety representatives and safety officers, and searches of manuscript and secondary literature on various joint gas management/union committees at regional and national level have all been used. These sources contain a wide selection of material, ranging from workers' accounts of work experiences in the gas industry before mechanization, through official records of national joint negotiation on health and safety and records of regional gas boards, relating to health and safety practices to interviews with senior managers in British Gas.

The gas industry had occupational hazards which were relatively well-researched in pre-nationalization days, and it is possible to make some assessment of occupational health information impacts on the workforce and relate this to workplace and trade union organization and the recommendations and actions of occupational physicians, employers and government agencies.

Some study qualifications

Industries, and indeed companies within industries, and plants within companies, vary considerably in their health and safety activity and effectiveness. There may be differences in employer and employee perceptions of health and safety's industrial relations importance (Batstone, Boraston and

Frenkel 1978; Edwards and Scullion 1982). Some industrial sectors and plants will have better health and safety records than others; some will have more occupational physicians and effective safety committees than others. Differences in the ways that professional groups like physicians, engineers and scientists tackle occupational health hazards may have industrial relations ramifications.

Production engineers may be more committed to production requirements because of their training, job descriptions and professional codes; physicians and research scientists may not face day-to-day production pressures and may have tighter ethical guidance on dealing with potential occupational health problems (Bayer 1988:3–11).

The gas industry cannot be assumed to be typical of all UK industry during the period in question. This case study, therefore, simply casts some light on aspects of those occupational health policies and practices of the period. The gas industry contained many hundreds of enterprises in the early years, which merit individual studies to assess the particular methods of handling health and safety disputes.

State and parliamentary activities on hazards at work provide a valuable, if limited, part of the picture of health and safety and industrial relations. MPs' and civil servants' debates and reports on factory legislation are useful, but do not provide any insight into what actually happened in the workplace and are one dimension of a multi-dimensional picture. Likewise, studies of national activity of trade unions, employers and managers on health and safety in the gas industry, although providing us with important evidence and impressions of experiences of occupational hazards, fail to give a very complete or coherent analysis of what precisely was happening in the workplace and why.

The gas industry, with its white, male, manual engineering workers in the period in question, would not represent a typical group of workers taking action on hazards in the 1990s. Studies of the health and safety organization and disputes which have involved women workers, non-trade unionists and black workers have been relatively rare (Watterson 1982, 1986).

The history of health hazards in the gas industry

In 1909, the gas industry consisted of 500 private companies and 292 local authorities working under statutory monopoly powers conferred, either by an Act of Parliament or a Provisional Order. A few local authorities and over 800 small gas companies produced gas without these powers. The workforce of the gas industry (production, distribution and service) was estimated at 80,000 in 1907 (Popplewell 1912:145–146).

Town gas was originally made through coal distillation and the original gasifiers were either vertical or horizontal retorts: the most hazardous retort for certain toxic gases, from the operators point of view, was the horizontal retort which was developed first, widely used in Britain, and which exposed workers to high fume levels well into the 1960s.

Medical evidence on health hazards

Considerable data on the hazards of the coal gas industry have now been collected (IARC 1984:82–99). Deelman, in 1923, found tar from horizontal gas retorts to be carcinogenic in mice, more rapidly than those from vertical retort houses. Doll, in 1965, found that death rates from lung cancer and bronchitis were highest in those gas workers most heavily exposed in the retorts, and lowest in those with no exposure. Retort-house operators apparently did not smoke more than other workers (IARC 1984:88). Henry, in 1931, had found elevated Standard Mortality Rates (SMRs hereafter) from bladder cancers for gas workers and in 1936 and 1947, Kennaway found elevated SMRs from lung cancer in gas stokers and coke over chargers, also in gas works engine drivers, gas works foremen, gas producers and gas fitters: gas stokers and coke oven chargers also had excess SMRs for laryngeal cancers (IARC 1984:90).

The retort house was the main method of gas production in the early part of the twentieth century and the carbonizing process used was one which entailed 24 hours production. The three key groups of gas workers were the 'Retort-house men', the 'Yardmen' and the 'Outside men'; the former group constituted a third of the total gas workforce. The introduction of machinery during the nineteenth century helped to lighten the workload of stokers, but nevertheless the jobs of retort-house operators and yardmen remained physically demanding and occupationally hazardous. Gas production was increased significantly in the 1880s, primarily through speed-ups and increased work pressure.

Between 1890 and 1910, profound changes occurred in the industry linked to 'the almost complete supersession of hand labour by machinery and mechanical devices generally' (Popplewell 1912:148–175; Hobsbawn 1968:158–178). Manual stoking machines were introduced in the 1890s and so too were mechanical conveyors for the transference of coal from yard to retort-house, and coke from retort-house to yard.

Employer evidence on health hazards

Despite these changes, retort-house operators, stokers and firemen still had heavy workloads in fume-filled gas works. One of the major arguments used by the 'new unions' in the late 1880s and early 1890s to support the introduction of the eight hour day, was that:

> there is an especial need for it [the eight hour day] in those industries where the conditions are dangerous or unhealthy, and that it would be generally desirable on physical and moral grounds (Royal Commission on Labour 1893–4:305; Radice and Radice 1974:20–29).

The gas employers, represented by the Incorporated Gas Institute, maintained in this same period that their industry was a healthy and safe one where, because directors of gas companies knew fit old gas workers, there was no need to produce and collate health statistics for the industry. The argument is, of course, fallacious because the health of the industry could only be assessed by looking at the numbers of gas workers who were ill of had died and therefore would not be seen by their former employers.

Worker evidence on health hazards

The non-scientific approach of the industry to occupational mortality and morbidity did not convince the gas workers' trade unions, although the Gas, Light and Coke Company produced a half yearly report from their consulting physician, George Hastings, which indicated that Metropolitan Gas Workers were only marginally less healthy than the Metropolitan Police force. The report fails to take account of the well-known, known now not then, confounding factor that has invalidated so many epidemiological studies which apparently show that there are no health risks to workers in a particular industry: namely the 'healthy worker' effect. In short, only relatively fit workers could become gas workers in the first place; so initially they would be healthier than the general population. When gas workers became ill, they often had to leave the gas industry and would not necessarily show up in that industry's morbidity and mortality figures. Such studies often failed to pick up the illnesses contracted by gas workers after they had retired, but such illnesses could be occupationally related.

The lack of accurate, systematically-collected statistics on gas workers' health creates a problem in assessing the health and safety record of the gas industry at this time. There is some evidence that chest diseases, particularly amongst stokers, were high, as well as evidence of an unusually high incidence of liver cancer, but these figures may simply reflect the hazards of the gas worker's general environment, rather than the work environment. What is beyond doubt, is that gas works at this time were hot, dusty and fume-filled places where men often 'took their meals close to ammonia and tar pumps with a gutter filled with liquid running close by' (Royal Commission 1893–4:29). We now know that those industries which have high fume and dust levels often tend to have excesses of lung and stomach diseases and those using tars and oil tend to have dermatitis problems. These sorts of problems were not uncommon in nineteenth and early twentieth century gas workers.

After much mechanization in 1912, an informed commentator on the gas industry still observed that 'the conditions as to temperature remain and only men of muscle and physique can stand the strain of retort-house work' (Popplewell 1912:157). In the same period, research in Berlin, Copenhagen, Magdeburg and Vienna revealed higher than average morbidity and mortality rates for all gas workers when compared with other occupational groups in those towns. Respiratory disease was particularly prevalent among gas workers.

This research was available to British gas workers in the 1920s through international trade union publications and shows that several European doctors perceived the hazards of the Victorian gas industry in a very different way to UK employers. The research also indicated that gas workers or their officials in Britain were well-informed about the hazards of the gas industry. The figures from the European report are in stark contrast to those offered by the London gas companies in the 1880s and may help to explain the scepticism shown by some gas workers in Britain during the 1920s and 1930s to the constant assurances from employers on the healthy state of their industry. Professor Loriga of Rome pointed out the health problems created by the contaminants in non-purified gas and the fume hazards in the purification problem in the 1920s:

> Feeding furnaces is very exhausting work because the workmen breathe coal dust and are also seriously affected by the heat ... Cleaning fire bars is always dangerous and unhealthy when it is done by hand. This is particularly the case when combustion goes on in the retort which allows fumes and gases to be inhaled. Other dangerous operations are the cleaning of smoke flues; and repairing fractures in retorts. Mass coke from horizontal and inclined retorts has to be drawn sometimes with a rake in works where machines are not used. Conveying, quenching and emptying retorts may be regarded as most unhealthy and dangerous in the gas making process (Loriga 1928:2).

Information on hazards was a prerequisite for any effective workplace health and safety action. The gas workers recognized the polluted nature of their environment but, like the scientists of the time, lacked the knowledge to identify precisely which pollutants were damaging them. Later work has since revealed that polycyclic aromatic hydrocarbons in gas production presented a major occupational cancer danger (Doll *et al.* 1965, 1972; Case 1975).

The chronology of gas hazard recognition is also important in the analysis of trade union, employer and medical response to workplace health and safety. The initial general impression given by the first two groups in the scientific and medical literature during the late nineteenth and early twentieth centuries, is that health and safety problems were either non-existent or of very little concern to the workers. Sources reveal that this impression is inaccurate for gas workers in the same period. Trade unionists like Will Thorne, commentators on labour like Frank Popplewell and worker advisers like Professor Loriga all described the hazards of dust and fumes faced by gas workers in the mechanized town gas industry.

Government evidence on health hazards

During the 1940s, new and more specific hazards were identified in the industry. In 1948, the General Register Office compiled a confidential report which stated that the makers of coal gas, coke and by-products (excluding tar distilling) had a mean annual death rate caused by tumours of the bladder, for the years 1945–47, over three times the average death rate for males over 14 in England and Wales (378 per million compared with 118 per million). A medical research worker investigating bladder tumours in retort-house workers during 1949 made the following observations on both vertical and horizontal retort working conditions:

> The general hazards in a retort house are 1. Minute dust from coal and coke. 2. Tar risks from tar deposits. 3. Coal gas which escapes from open and leaking valves. At some undertakings many sources of leak were present, ventilation was bad and raw coal gas fumes pervaded the whole house, whereas in other works the retort houses were extremely airy and a negative pressure was kept in the pipes at any sign of a leak. The vertical retorts and therefore the fumes are more concentrated than the horizontal. [When stokers either cleared the off-takes or ensured the coal was travelling through the retort, they were exposed to raw coal gas.] I am told that new stokers cough and splutter when doing these jobs but old hands develop a knack of avoiding the fumes as much as possible. However, I feel it is inevitable that considerable quantities would be inhaled in the course of a day's work and that much would condense on the men's clothing and hands. Depending on the Construction of the works and the direction of the wind, fumes may reach other men not employed in the retort house and it must be remembered that the whole plan and arrangement of many of the undertakings has been radically changed since the commencement date of employment of the men concerned (Kosker 1975:16–17).

Recognition of hazards and potential hazards was not restricted to 'expert' researchers in the field, but came much earlier through workers and, in some instances, their representatives too (Table 1). The extent to which individual employers and employers federations received, digested and disseminated this information is difficult to assess.

Table 1 Gas retort-house workers and cancer: A history of GMBATU worker and scientific knowledge

A Gas worker knowledge

1920/1	GMWU representatives at Gas NJIC ask employers for an enquiry into deaths and disease amongst gas workers especially 'top men' on retort houses. Employers say records inadequate to do this.
1929	GMWU officials in Nottingham circulate Public Service Employees' Federation report on gas industry pitch cancers – employers dismiss it.
1938	TUC Medical Advisor sends GMWU evidence on lung and digestive problems in gas workers.
1944	Birmingham Region GMWU refers problems of fumes from retort houses to a Worcester GP via a member's case.
1946/7	GMWU delegates at Conference raise problems of bronchitis and appalling conditions in retort houses. Union journal carries article on adverse effects of coal gas.
1956	Doll sends GMWU National Officer his report on lung cancer in gas workers.
1962	GMWU Scottish Region win one bladder case of compensation for bladder cancer from DHSS for a gas worker using the disease that was prescribed following the rubber industry cancer tragedy.
1975	TGWU win £4,500 tort compensation against Southern Gas for kidney cancer in retort worker, using Case's evidence.

B Scientific knowledge

1906	Skin cancer from pitch and tar covered by Compensation Acts.
1924	Kennaway discovers tar carcinogens in gas works.
1931	Henry and Kennaway show excess bladder cancer in gas and tar distillation workers.
1933/9	Coal tar and pitch found to contain alpha and betanaphthylamine which were known to cause bladder cancer in the dyestuffs industry.
1947	Kennaway shows excess lung cancer in gas workers.
1948	Report from General Registry Office confirm coal gas workers had three times expected bladder cancer rate.
1952	Doll reports on coal carbonization workers who have lung cancer risk.
1956	Doll sends GMWU National his report on lung cancer in gas.
1958	Registrar General's Office Report for 1949–53 showed that makers of coal gas and coke had twice the expected rate of bladder cancer.
1965	Doll studies gas boards and concludes that retort-house work causes lung cancer and bronchitis.
1975	Doll's further studies lead him to conclude that bladder and lung cancer are caused by work both on horizontal and vertical retort houses.

Source: Gee and Watterson, 1988.

Formal structures for dealing with or 'ducking' industrial disease questions: worker and medical action and employer responses on gas hazards in the early twentieth century

In 1919, a Whitley Council National Joint Industrial Council (hereafter NJIC) was established for bargaining between gas employers and the Gas Workers Union. Prior to this date, gas companies had used profit-sharing schemes and co-partnership projects as a method of excluding independent Trade Unions and maintaining company unions (Clegg 1954:152, 160). Unions like the GMWU had to talk to the 1,200 gas producing undertakings individually. The first formally agreed function of the Gas NJIC was to consider 'the wages, hours and working conditions in the industry as a whole'; its second function was to consider the means of maximizing production and employment; its third function was to settle disputes, and its fourth function was 'the improvement of the health conditions obtaining in the industry and the provision of special treatment, where necessary, for workers in the industry' (Williamson 1939:101–119).

In 1921 the NJIC proposed a Joint Works Committee Model Constitution which referred to 'improving and ameliorating working conditions', including questions relating to the health and safety of the workpeople. However, very few such committees were ever formed. The change in attitudes of employers and trade unions to the various consultative bodies between 1920 and 1940 is illustrative of the national pattern of political change.

Trade union actions and employer responses

The Gas NJIC made several references to the hazards of the industry in the 1920s and 1930s and showed some concern about working conditions. Employees requested data from the employers on the death rate of gas workers prior to the introduction of vertical gas retorts and after the new methods of gas carbonization came in during the late 1920s. The GMWU worker representatives reported complaints from the 'top men' on the vertical retorts relating to high fumes and temperature levels. The employers confessed such requests would be difficult to accede to, because illness records in the past were very fragmentary and incomplete, and comparisons would be most misleading, but they were willing to ascertain the 'actual facts' (NJIC 10th Annual Report 1928–9:7). Any worker request for health and safety information involved employers in the expenditure of time and money and therefore, in the short-term, affected profits to a lesser or greater extent.

The gas employers' response in 1928 contrasts significantly with the industry view of the 1890s, when firm assurances were given about the absence of risk in the industry and the fullness of statistical information. As Professor Robert Case has pointed out, however:

> There would have been reason to be aware since at the latest 1907 that one form of cancer was an occupational hazard in occupations where coal tar was encountered, and reason since 1931 to believe that cancer of the bladder should now so be regarded. Subsequent periodical 'monitoring' of the gas industry in the reports from the Registrar-General consistently supported this viewpoint (Case 1975:22–23).

Sir Ernest Kennaway identified a risk of bladder cancer in 1931 among coal production workers. Gas works chemists should have known, at the latest in 1933, that alpha- and betanaphthylamine (the carcinogens of the bladder) were produced in gas retorts. These facts are important in considering gas employer responses on the NJIC during 1928/9 to workers requests for information and further investigation of the subject.

Employers must have been aware of the typical conditions in their industry and the degree to which their workforce might be exposed either to tar or to fumes containing carcinogens. Herbert Mannion, a gas worker in the inter-war years, gives a graphic account of his job charging retorts:

> The place is now filled with the coal dust and breeze from the coke which is hot when it falls on our faces, arms and chests. As one retort-cover after another is opened, the atmosphere becomes poisonous with sulphur; heavy smoke pours out of the retorts before they can be closed, making the place pitch-black ... Smoke rises to the roof slowly and more of it rushes from out of the charged and uncharged retorts: an infernal mixture of crude gas, sulphur, smoke and tar, enough to suffocate a whole regiment of soldiers. Our eyes are full of coal-dust, frantically we wipe them with our sweat rags; breeze, dust, and God knows-what-else gets up our noses, into our mouths; we cough and splutter and sneeze – truly, this is the shift of shifts! (Each shift did ten firings of the retort) ...... Sweating, taking breath with difficulty in the mixture of steam and 'smuge' from the top of the stack like devils in Hell we carry on till the last fire is full (Mannion 1938:157–159).

The gas workers again raised the question of occupational ill-health and the hazards of pitch tar in 1938. Yet there is no reference by the gas manufacturers to bladder cancer risks, the work of industrial chemists and Kennaway on amines in retort houses or of any other health and safety issue, for that matter, between 1920 and 1944.

Employer inaction – despite, in Case's opinion, the fact that the industry had knowledge of the skin cancer hazards in gas production in 1907 and bladder cancer in 1931 – contrasts starkly with worker calls for action. These calls came through the formal structure of the NJIC and National Office of the GMWU, and probably emanated from the lay members. In

1929, the Gas Workers Union, the GMWU, was aware of the higher mortality of gas workers in Europe and some parts of the union had particular worries. The Midland Region of the GMWU was particularly concerned about the new carbonization processes in the 1920s and 1930s and wanted an ILO survey of hazards in gas production. In addition to the European reports on hazards (NJIC GMWU Ms. Minutes, 1929, 1/19/1), the union knew that in Dortmund in 1927 Professor B. Chajes had referred to the dangers of smoke, fumes and gas in coke and gas works and the high incidence of cancer in the same group of workers (GMWU Mss 1927/8,1/19/3).

The Medical Adviser to the TUC, Dr Morgan, produced a report on sulphur poisoning and examined not just sulphur dioxide and carbon monoxide poisoning but other gases like hydrogen sulphide and the by-products of tar produced in coal gas manufacture. Morgan knew of German work on the industry's hazards and also referred to Austrian and Danish evidence on the above average incidences of respiratory diseases and digestive problems of gas workers in his report (GMWU Ms. 1938 1/19/4).

Limits of formal trade union action on hazards

From 1938 to 1965 there were no further references to occupational health in the NJIC minutes, although certain developments did take place behind the scenes. In the 1930s, the TUC produced a pamphlet on dermatitis in industry and in 1935 numerous dermatitis cases were reported by gas workers exposed to tar and paints in GMWU Districts. In 1938, London gas workers called for action on pitch and tar but by the mid-1940s, the union complaints about dermatitis had declined significantly (GMWU Ms. 1/19/2).

In 1944, the Social Insurance Department of the TUC began an investigation into the harmful effects of dust and fumes in a range of industries, and informed the GMWU of the work. There are no details about any union follow-up, although Tom Williamson, the GMWU National Gas Officer, received the papers on the subject. In July 1944, Williamson had been contacted by the Joint Manager of the Federation of Gas Employers in London on a similar issue. The Company had been informed that a Worcester GP was carrying out an investigation, allegedly for the GMWU, on the effects of fumes and coke dust on men working in the Worcester retort house and gas works. The company manager observed that:

> it is unfortunate, to say the least of it, if in Wartime any of your Union Officials are taking action such as is alleged. As you know conditions are abnormal, but I am sure that Engineers throughout the country are doing everything possible to improve conditions (GMWU NJIC Ms. 1944, 1/19/1).

The union at a national level may well have been unaware of this case but it is generally true to state that, at the time, health and safety had a low priority with many British national union officials for a variety of reasons. Compensation rather than hazard removal was probably the most that workers expected at the time. Even then, however, there were many difficulties. The Worcester GMWU Branch Secretary who worked in the gas industry, had been certified a pneumoconiosis sufferer, but the gas industry lay outside this scheme for the purposes of workmen's compensation. Charles Dukes of the GMWU raised the matter and contacted the TUC to pressurize for additions to the appropriate schedule. The member's own doctor had suggested to the GMWU Midland District Secretary that it would help the case if data could be obtained on the subject, and had so started his own enquiry. The letter from the employers' side revealed a considerable sensitivity on the subject and the minutes of the NJIC in the previous decades revealed no interest and no action reported by the employers.

These events do not indicate a low-risk industry with quiescent workers, nor ineffective union officials satisfied with working conditions. The pressure for improvements on health and safety increased at the GMWU's Annual Congress in 1946 when gas workers called for chronic bronchitis to be placed on the prescribed industrial disease schedule.

In 1947 and 1949 lay members of the same union, also at Congresses, openly criticized the appalling conditions in retort houses and gas purification plants (GMWU Congress Reports 1950, 1954). In 1950 the GMWU received details from, and attended the International Conference for Employees in the Gas and Electricity Industries in Blackpool. Occupational illnesses of gas workers were raised and the Conference wanted details of preventive health measures taken to safeguard gas workers (GMWU Ms. 1951, 1/19/3). Criticisms of the gas industry were made during the transitional period of nationalization in Britain: the Gas Act reached the statute book in 1948 and the new structures, particularly on health and safety, worked their way through from 1950 onwards.

Sir Richard Doll's pioneering paper on increased risks of lung cancer deaths in gas workers appeared in the *British Journal of Industrial Medicine* in 1952. Two years earlier, a gas worker had criticized conditions of work in British industry, called for general health and safety improvements in the country and, at the GMWU's Congress of 1954, raised the question of gas workers' particular susceptibility to lung cancer. The worker wanted an investigation of the disease amongst gas workers and a joint committee of inquiry with the Union and Gas Council (GMWU Congress Reports 1950, 1954). Nothing happened until 1956 when Sir Fred Heyday, the GMWU National Gas Officer, contacted Doll and asked for his paper on lung cancer, which Heyday had heard about from a TUC General Council colleague at the Gas NJIC. Doll complied with the request in July 1956 (GMWU Ms. 1/19/5/A).

Closing the stable door ... the familiar consequences of neglecting industrial diseases

The problems of occupational cancer, especially bladder and lung cancer, and the gas workers lingered on. The gas industry hazards raised by workers and scientists in the 1920s and 1930s were still unresolved in the 1960s. In September 1962, the *Daily Express* reported the continuing existence of an above average incidence of cancer in gas workers. Lay gas members of the GMWU in the Athol gas station in Liverpool raised the matter with their District Secretary who in turn yet again contacted the union's National Gas Officer, Sir Fred Heyday. He responded by telling the Liverpool members that he was unaware of the press reports on the hazard, but that several years ago the union had investigated the subject when Doll's work showed tar irritants in gas work air were the cause of slightly increased gas cancer rates! (GMWU Ms. 1962, 1/19/5). No action appeared to have been taken at the national level of the union at this time despite Dr Murray, the TUC's Medical Adviser, sending Heyday a copy of Doll's 1965 article from the *British Journal of Industrial Medicine*. The article revealed further evidence of the health risks run by gas workers.

The gas workers themselves continued to highlight the hazards they faced, in spite of the apparent reluctance by their national officer to get involved in any formal action. In 1959, three years before the Liverpool workers were to call for an enquiry, the Canning Town Engineering Branch had proposed at the GMWU Congress that the NEC should do all they could to get chest complaints and bronchitis in gas workers prescribed as an industrial disease. These gas workers, cited, firstly, evidence of chest troubles in gas workers gathered by Dr Harris Jones at the Middlesex Hospital in 1959 and, secondly, the mortality rate of vertical gas house operators who were unusually largely recruited from fit ex-guardsmen and, thirdly, evidence collected in 1954 from the Compensation Department in Liverpool. The union called for further information, not action on the matter (GMWU Congress Report 1959).

The tragic consequences of exposure to retort-house fumes was fully revealed in the GMWU's journal of 1963, following a report in *The Scotsman* of January that year, when a bladder cancer fatality was recorded in a gas worker. In 1960 a Scottish retort-house worker had died of bladder cancer which his surgeon believed was occupationally caused. The union claimed state compensation but this was initially rejected by the insurance officer. After medical evidence had been submitted on the effects of betanaphthylamine and coal tar in the gas industry, the Ministry of Health finally accepted the claim, but said it would only consider future cases on an individual basis (GMWU Journal, 1963:2).

Doll's last paper on coal carbonizing plant workers was published in 1972 and he confirmed the increased risk of bladder and lung cancer for those working in or near vertical and horizontal retort houses. In 1975 a gas retort worker finally received £4,500 for an occupationally contracted kidney cancer. The judge concluded that gas employers should have been aware of hazards in the industry and taken steps to eliminate them when the retort operator was at work.

Gas production technology has moved on and there are no longer operational gas retort houses across the country. There are, however, still significant numbers of retort-house workers in the 1990s who have worked with the old technology and who may have contracted occupationally-related disease. Knowledge about their occupational disease claims is limited and it appears likely that many in the 1980s and 1990s did not get compensation for their illnesses.

The political economy of occupational disease in the gas industry

The reasons for the failure of union full-time officers to gain compensation and remedial action for the gas workers in the first part of the twentieth century are not totally clear. Factors may have included the nature and purpose of the NJIC; the lack of knowledge of the union full-time officers on hazards; a combination of attitudes to health and safety which accorded the subject low priority on union 'shopping lists'. Occupational safety and related production issues were short-term, tangible subjects more easily dealt with by union officials familiar with wage bargaining issues than long-term industrial disease prevention campaigns. Similarly, trade union efforts to obtain industrial injury compensation for members were relatively easier to manage for a full-time officer than dealing with occupational illnesses and getting an industrial disease prescribed.

Several health risks of the gas industry were ignored in the NJIC between the 1940s and 1960s, and instead the body considered organization of safety committees (1949), overalls and protective clothing (1949), sick pay and injury procedures (1961–2), conditions payments (1967), natural gas safety (1970) and the hazards of electrical cables for gas road workers (1970). The only major hazard dealt with between 1945 and 1976 was that of asbestos where information was gained from the TUCCIOH (TUC Centenary Institute of Occupational Health) and the unions pressed for asbestos substitutes, masks and a Code of Practice on the material (GMWU NJIC Ms. 1976/1453). The NJIC seemed to have a limited effect on health and safety between 1945 and the early 1970s: issues which employers wished to ignore were apparently usually ignored. The health and safety issues raised, tended to relate to production requirements, safety clothing – which emphasized worker responsibility for accidents and illnesses at work – and compensation issues. Even here, formal questions of compensation for lung and bladder cancer were apparently not raised at the NJIC by the unions until the 1970s.

The unions in the gas industry (primarily the GMWU and TGWU) were not inactive on health and safety outside the NJIC. In 1977, the GMWU and TGWU with British Gas, ICI and the British rubber industry funded the Royal Marsden Hospital Cancer Project which looked at a range of occupations involved in bladder cancer cases (NJIC Gas File 1/19/1).

With the passage of the Health and Safety at Work Act (HASAWA) in 1974 the GMWU examined its health and safety organization and then began to look more closely at the potential role of safety representatives and the value of safety committees in effecting health and safety improvements at the workplace.

Informal worker action on hazards

There is no record of any official stoppage on a gas health and safety issue between 1920 and 1970. This does not show that there were no disputes, but simply that there were no officially recorded strikes (Department of Employment Manuscript Books; Watterson 1988:193–258). In the records of nineteenth century gas works, there are occasional accounts of strife. In 1888 at the New Street gas works in Edinburgh, stokers protested about their working conditions to the Edinburgh Commissioners and complained of excessive heat from the four ovens in the eight retorts and called for the operation of only three ovens, otherwise they would strike; the threat was sufficient to get an agreement from management to improve conditions (Thompson 1953:28).

The campaigns for shorter working hours in the nineteenth century have been much under-estimated for their contribution to health and safety, because reduced hours reduced the exposure of workers to dust and fumes; health, safety and welfare are in a sense an implicit and integral part of any trade union campaign to reduce the working week. The lack of strike action in an industry full of hazards might indicate the powerful control the employers exercised in the labour market relationships with the potential workforce: perhaps further enhanced by the policy in some regions of recruiting mainly ex-Guards Regiment workers into retort houses. This ploy certainly did not produce a passive workforce in those regions. But the impact of the economic depressions and the failure of the General Strike weakened all trade unionists in the 1920s and 1930s in their efforts to improve conditions by industrial action.

Gas companies had well-established paternalist traditions, epitomized by the Metropolitan Gas Company welfare and accident committees and the profit-sharing programmes and anti-trade union schemes which operated in other gas companies before 1919. These developments had something in common with the schemes operated by Renold's in Manchester and the Rowntree and Cadbury's factories, as well as the policies of a number of American companies in the 1920s and 1930s. After 1919, the NJIC served to focus trade union activity on health and safety issues and then neutralize that interest. Despite trade union opposition at a local level to consultative committees, the NJIC did very little, if any, negotiation on hazards, preferring what appears to have been a desultory form of behind the scenes consultation with employers on the subject.

In theory, eleven regional councils of the NJIC existed to discuss wages, hours and conditions. In practice, the Federation of Gas Employers (established in 1919 but originating in the National Gas Council established in 1916 and the Institute of Gas Engineers established in 1863) maintained control of the machinery. Many companies set up co-partnership schemes to neutralize worker action, in some cases including worker representatives on the Board of Directors (Chantler, 1938:32–33). Thompson found that after 1920 in the Scottish gas industry, little worked well in the field of consultation except the Canteen and Safety Committee in Edinburgh. Here the safety committee had no budget and the worker members were nominated by management, who for their part, thought the safety committee worked well (Thompson:367).

There are dangers in trying to read history selectively and the gas industry may well not have been typical of other industries at the time. However, the gas industry does appear to fall in the category of Whitley Council industries

> associated with diluted bargaining industries and other areas of employment with weak union organisation [where it was common] to find joint consultation grafted on top of these arrangements (Ramsay, 1980:385).

World War II, with its emphasis on production, saw a resurgence of interest in joint consultation, a policy which had never waned in the gas industry. In 1943 there were no fewer than 4,169 Joint Production Committees established, covering two million workers in British industry and able to discuss efficiency and production, but not matters covered by the negotiating machinery (Ramsay 1980:388). Between 1950 and 1965, the dangers of lung cancer, bladder cancer and bronchitis had all been identified in retort-house workers and yet, except in the West Midlands Research Centre, no time was apparently devoted to the subject in official reports. One wonders what the response of the industry would have been if the public had run a similar risk to the retort-house operators and had received information to that effect?

An analysis of health and safety issues

The explanations for inaction on health hazards in the early twentieth century gas industry are complex and relate to a wide range of factors prevailing at the time. Crudely put, there was an obvious conflict between production and productivity on the one hand, and health and safety on the other hand, in terms of resources, time and knowledge. How this worked out in practice was a very complex process indeed. Attitudes varied from region to region and group to group but emanated from explicit and implicit values within industry, the socialization of managers and workers before and after entering the gas industry, the weight of national campaigns, the balance of power between capital and labour, the relatively low status given to occupational health in the UK, the control of the use of occupational medical knowledge by the state and employers, the dominance of the medical model in occupational health and the lack of interest in or downright hostility to occupational health education in the workplace for much of this time (Watterson 1986; Watterson 1990).

The gas industry was known for its hot, dusty and fume-filled work well into the 1960s. The research of Ms Hosker, Case's assistant in the 1975 bladder cancer case, revealed that standards in gas works did vary considerably and some were well-ventilated and well-maintained establishments. However, industry standards tended to reflect the average or less good works rather than the better works. The wider social factors – workers' expectations, factory inspectors' expectations, local, family and school adjustment to and acceptance of industries which had 'traditions' of certain types of poor working conditions – were important influences on worker action or adjustment to low health and safety standards.

The environmental factors linked to the state of the local labour market – with very limited job choices for working-class kids – led many working in dirty, dangerous industries to accept, at least initially, the existence of those conditions as normal and unchangeable. It is therefore surprising that, in some respects, gas workers in the GMWU did demonstrate their concern about health hazards from the 1920s through to the 1960s.

Conclusion

Gas workers recognized some of the occupational disease hazards in their industry in the late nineteenth and early twentieth centuries. Worker epidemiology picked up hazards in coal gas production and, where it could, incorporated research from mainstream epidemiology and occupational medicine. The gas workers struggled against, and indeed wrote accounts of, their working conditions to combat the social construction of ignorance about occupational ill-health in their industry. Nevertheless, the gas workers were, in terms of Turner's sociology of occupational disease, neither able to alter the dominant established social processes for defining occupational diseases, nor overcome the political economy of the time which created particular gas industry health hazards.

Demands for preventive action against hazards and compensation for workers adversely affected, emerged from lay trade unionists in the early part of the twentieth century. Despite this, the political economy of the gas industry and the social processes – not necessarily of constituting diseases related to gas production but rather of bringing these diseases to the attention of those at risk and compensating them – were sufficiently powerful to thwart those demands. In terms of conflicting professional groups, the work of the few toxicologists and epidemiologists who identified the occupational diseases related to coal gas production, was never able to overcome the economic and political power of the gas companies and the government departments controlling the regulation of health and safety and compensation schemes for industrial diseases between the late 1890s and the 1960s.

Occupational medicine lost the struggle to political economy at an early date. None of Legge's four basic occupational health axioms in 1934 were fully implemented. The gas industry at the time did not do everything it could to protect retort-house workers at risk; removal of hazards at source and engineering controls of dust and fumes were not introduced across the industry; and workers were still not told of the hazards of working on retort houses well after those hazards had been documented in the scientific literature.

The ability of the gas industry's consultative mechanisms to turn worker health and safety concerns into meetings about productivity, efficiency and safety flag awards was considerable. This transformation was achieved through an elaborate structure of joint consultative committees, local joint industrial councils and regional joint industrial councils (Gas NJIC minutes and gas regional reports). Many of the obstacles to improved health and safety identified in Codrington and Henley's study of the construction industry are becoming commonplace and now exist in the gas industry. They include problems with weak union organization, economic recession, the impact of sub-contractors and privatization with all that potentially entails for health and safety standards.

By the time the serious occupational hazards in the industry had been identified, officially recognized and accepted for the purposes of prescribed industrial disease benefit, technology had moved on to new gas production processes and new potential hazards. The risks to gas workers in the pre-natural gas period were not as high as those in mining, chemicals and foundries but nevertheless they were substantial and affected the retort-house workers, to a high degree. Now the health hazards of natural gas are less and there are far fewer production workers. Detailed research on natural gas processing hazards, however, is not widely available and some gas workers are still exposed to potentially toxic chemicals.

The story is not unique: similar tales exist for asbestos workers, plastics workers, textile workers – with mule spinners cancer and byssinosis, welders and foundry workers with respiratory diseases, engineering workers with vibration-induced white finger, shipbuilders with occupational deafness, data processors with repetitive strain injuries ... and so on.

References

Bagnara, S., Misiti, R. and Wintersberger, H. (eds), (1985), *Work and Health in the 1980s*, Bonn: Sigma Edition.

Batstone, E., Boraston, I. and Frenkel, S. (1978), *The Social Organisation of Strikes*, Oxford: Basil Blackwell.

Bayer, R. (ed.) (1988), *The Health and Safety of Workers: Case Studies in the Politics of Personal Responsibility*, Oxford: Oxford University Press.

Berman, D. (1978), *Death on the Job*, New York: Monthly Review Press.

British Gas Annual Reports 1972/3 to 1979/80.

British Gas Regional Annual Reports 1970 to 1980.

Brown, P. (ed.) (1989), *Perspectives in Medical Sociology*, Belmont, California: Wadsworth.

Carson, W.G. (1981), *The Other Price of Britain's Oil*, Oxford: Martin Robertson.

Case R.A.M. (1975), Manuscript Notes on British Gas Corporation Kidney Cancer Compensation Case.

Chantler, P. (1938), *The British Gas Industry*, Manchester: Manchester University Press.

Clegg, H. (1954), *The General Union*, Oxford: Basil Blackwell.

Codrington, C. and Henley, J. (1981), 'The industrial relations of industry and death: safety representatives in the construction industry', *British Journal of Industrial Relations*, **19**:297–315.

Creighton, B. and Gunningham, N. (eds) (1985), *The Industrial Relations of Occupational Health and Safety*, Sydney: Croom Helm.

Dawson, S., Willman, P., Bamford, M. and Clinton, C. (1988), *Safety at Work: the Limits of Self-Regulation*, Cambridge: Cambridge University Press.

Doll, R. (1952), 'The causes of death among gas workers with particular reference to cancer of the lung', *British Journal of Industrial Medicine*, **9**:180–185.

Doll, R., Fisher, R.W. and Gammon, E.J. (1965), 'Mortality of gas workers with special reference to cancers of the lung and bladder, chronic bronchitis and pneumoconiosis', *British Journal of Industrial Medicine*, **22**:1–12.

Doll, R., Vessey, M.P. and Beasley, R.W. (1972), 'The mortality of gas workers:

final report of a prospective study', *British Journal of Industrial Medicine*, **29**:394–406.
Edwards, P.K. and Scullion, H. (1982), *The Social Organisation of Industrial Conflict*, Oxford: Basil Blackwell.
Elling, R.H. (1986), *The Struggle for Workers Health: a Study of Six Industrialised Countries*, New York: Baywood.
The Gas Act 1948, London: HMSO.
The Gas Act 1972, London: HMSO.
General and Municipal Workers Union, Gas Industry Health and Safety Manuscript Papers, GMBATU Head Office, London.
General and Municipal Workers Union (1920–1980), Biennial and Annual Congress Reports.
General and Municipal Workers Union, Journals 1945–1980.
Gersuny, C. (1981), *Work Hazards and Industrial Conflict*, Hanover and London: University Press of New England.
Gill, C., Morris, R. and Eaton, J. (1978), *Industrial Relations and the Chemical Industry*, Farnborough: Saxon House.
Hobsbawn, E.J. (1968), *Labouring Men*, London: Weidenfeld and Nicholson.
International Agency for Research on Cancer (1984), *IARC Monographs on the Evaluation of Carcinogenic Risk of Chemicals to Humans: Polycyclic Aromatic Compounds Part 3, Coal Gasification, Volume 34*, Lyons: IARC.
International Federation of Public Service Employees (1928), Report on the Hazards of the Gas Industry, mimeo.
Kosker, M. (1975), unpublished evidence recorded in the Case R.M., typescript.
Judkins, B.M. (1986), *We Offer Ourselves as Evidence: towards Worker Control of Occupational Health*, New York: Greenwood Press.
Labisch, A. (1985), 'The social history of occupational medicine and factory health services in the Federal Republic of Germany', in Weindling, P. (ed.), *The Social History of Occupational Health*, London: Croom Helm.
Legge, T. (1934), *Industrial Maladies*, London: Oxford University Press.
Loriga, G. (1928), *Industrial Accidents and Diseases in Gas and Electricity Undertakings*, Rome: ILO.
Mannion, H. (1938), 'I was in a gas works', in Common, J. (ed.) *Seven Shifts*, London: Secker and Warburg.
Morrison, J.G. (n.d.), The Safety Representative in the Gas Industry, mimeo.
National Joint Industrial Council Minute Books of the Gas Industry, held at GMB London Offices.
Navarro, V. and Berman, D.M. (1983), *Health and Work under Capitalism: An International Perspective*, New York: Baywood.
Nelkin, D. and Brown, M. (1984), *Workers at Risk: Voices from the Workplace*, Chicago: Chicago University Press.
Nelkin, D. (ed.) (1985), *The Language of Risk: Conflicting Perspectives on Occupational Health*, Beverly Hills: Sage.
Nichols, W.A.T. and Armstrong, P. (1973), *Safety or Profit*, Bristol: Falling Wall Press.
Otway, H. (1985), 'Regulation and risk analysis', in Otway, H. and Peltu, M. (eds), *Regulating Industrial Risks: Science, Hazards and Public Protection*, London: Butterworths.

Popplewell, F. (1912), 'The gas industry', in Webb, S. and Freeman, A. (eds) *Seasonal Trades by Various Writers*, London: Constable and Co.
Radice, E.A. and Radice, G.H. (1974), *Will Thorne*, London: Allen and Unwin.
Ramsay, H.A. (1980), 'Participation: the pattern and its significance', in Nichols, W.A.T. (ed.), *Capital and Labour*, Glasgow: Fontana.
Robson, W.A. (ed.) (1952), *Problems of Nationalised Industries*, London: Allen and Unwin.
Robson, W.A. (1960), *Nationalised Industries and Public Ownership*, London: Allen and Unwin.
Rowland, A. (1980), 'Tanning leather, tanning hides', *Radical America*, Nov/Dec: 23–37.
Royal Commission on Labour (1891–1894), Reports, Parliamentary Papers, London: HMSO.
Sallis, D. (1965), 'Joint consultations and meetings of primary working groups in power stations', *British Journal of Industrial Relations*, **111**:326–344.
Thompson, A.E. (1953), 'Industrial relations in the fuel and power industries with particular reference to selected undertakings in Midlothian', unpublished Ph.D. thesis, University of Edinburgh.
Turner, B.S. (1987), *Medical Knowledge and Social Power*, London: Sage Publications.
Watterson, A.E. (1982), 'American trade unions and health and safety: recent developments and past experiences', *The Industrial Tutor*, **3**:74–85.
Watterson, A.E. (1986), 'Occupational health and illness: the politics of hazards education', in Rodmell, S. and Watt, A. (eds), *The Politics of Health Education.*
Watterson, A.E. (1988), 'Industrial relations and health and safety at work in post-war Britain: a study of conflict and control in the workplace', unpublished Ph.D. thesis, Bristol University.
Watterson, A.E. (1990), 'Occupational health education in the United Kingdom workplace: looking backwards and going forwards?', *British Journal of Industrial Medicine*, **47**:366–371.
Weindling, P. (ed.) (1985), *The Social History of Occupational Health*, London: Croom Helm.
Williams, T.I. (1981), *A History of the British Gas Industry*, Oxford: Oxford University Press.
Williamson, T. (1939), 'The Joint Industrial Council and the municipal gas industry', in Gannett, F.E. and Catherwood, B.F. (eds), *Industrial and Labour Relations in Great Britain*, New York: P.S. King and Sons.

9 How do places shape health? Rethinking locality and lifestyle in North-East England

Peter Phillimore

Introduction

This is, in some ways, a speculative analysis. It suggests how far we still have to go to understand the social creation of health differentials. But behind it lies a disparity in health – between working class Middlesbrough and working class Sunderland – which is anything but speculative. The particular case to be discussed here graphically illustrates Benton's recent reminder that 'social and geographical differentials in environmental risks to health are only partially mapped by conventional measures of socio-economic inequality' (1991:6).

Analysis of the social distribution of health occupies a curious position in sociology – and even more so in social anthropology. At once of considerable importance in its potential for highlighting the cumulative consequences of social inequality, and with enormous ramifications for policy, the subject has nevertheless remained surprisingly marginal to wider debates about the sociological conceptualization and representation of social life. One reason must surely be that the debate around health inequalities, which has flourished anew since publication of the Black Report (DHSS 1980; Townsend and Davidson 1982), has been conducted first and foremost within an epidemiological paradigm. For all that sociologists have contributed to an understanding of these inequalities, the empirical cast of the debate has largely been dictated by the principles of measurement in epidemiology. Developments in the field have been shaped but also confined by the health and population data sets available (Benton 1991:6). This data-driven character has undoubtedly helped to make the debate about health inequalities seem unduly peripheral within sociology at large.

These limitations are plain to see in relation to the sub-field of geographic inequalities in health. For long the main alternative to a class-based approach, studies of health in small areas have flourished over the last decade, facilitated by the technical development of postcoding the officially registered life events of birth and death. The value of this genre of work has been real enough. Indeed, I suspect that locality has provided a more accessible and effective framework than occupational class for impressing on public awareness the full severity of health inequalities. Nevertheless, this kind of research rests upon an unsatisfactorily narrow range of data sources, in which the Census in effect represents the social. It is indicative that measures of deprivation, for instance, have generated much more interest among epidemiologists than they are likely to do among sociologists. The shortcomings of relying upon such limited data may in fact be masked in comparisons of health which span the whole social spectrum, for it is not hard to demonstrate clear associations between gross differentials in wealth and health (Carstairs and Morris 1989; Congdon 1988; Townsend *et al.* 1987, 1988), as a result making it seem less imperative to look beyond the parameters of the data already in use. Problems of limited data are much more likely to arise, on the other hand, in relation to apparent anomalies, and it is in such instances that the researcher is obliged to look beyond the convenience of routine data. I intend to explore this theme through a comparison between two large towns in north-east England, Middlesbrough and Sunderland. The chapter revolves around a contrast in mortality of puzzling magnitude. Why should mortality be so much higher in the poorer and predominantly working class areas of Middlesbrough than in areas of neighbouring Sunderland which are, on conventional measures, similarly poor? (Phillimore 1990; Phillimore and Morris 1991). I call this a puzzle advisedly, for there is very little in contemporary literature on British health inequalities to make us anticipate such a wide disparity between two such ostensibly similar populations. A derivative question is to ask whether there are insights to be gained from looking at other fields of sociological research: most obviously in relation to recent work on social and economic change in localities. The purpose here is to explore three themes, not easily turned into the kind of data set this field of research has always relied upon, which may nevertheless have a bearing on the mortality differentials which motivate the enquiry.

Premature mortality in Middlesbrough and Sunderland

What do these differentials amount to? Here I shall briefly summarize the background to this research, with certain key mortality statistics.

It was apparent from Townsend *et al.* (1988) that no other part of the Northern Region of England experienced such consistently high premature mortality in the early 1980s as the south bank of the River Tees. On the summary 'index of material deprivation' used in that study, made up of four variables derived from the 1981 Census, this area also emerged as extremely deprived. By contrast, similarly deprived areas of Sunderland also stood out, but for the opposite reason: premature mortality, although above the national average, appeared unexpectedly moderate. Three-year snapshots of mortality have their value, but in comparisons of this kind their limitations are apparent. It was decided to clarify whether or not the years 1981–83 were typical by analysing mortality over a much longer period, therefore, than was usual in small area studies of health. An extended sequence of 12 years was taken, from 1975 to 1986. Data on deaths were assembled for the entire area of both towns, although the prime interest was in comparison of the least affluent areas in each. To that end, two areas were identified which were considerably more deprived than anywhere else in either town. These areas were made up of 17 wards in Middlesbrough and 8 in Sunderland, with populations in 1981 of 100,000 and 92,000 respectively. In both places, these formed continuous tracts, broken only by the River Wear in Sunderland. On a set of core census indicators from the 1981 and the 1971 Censuses, these two zones were strikingly similar: both were and are at the extremity of deprivation within the region, although Middlesbrough probably had the edge in 1981. (For a fuller discussion of methods, see Phillimore and Morris 1991.)

Analysis over the 12 years 1975–86 confirms that death rates under the age of 65 have consistently been much greater in the selected areas of Middlesbrough than in Sunderland. Table 1 summarizes a few key statistics. Throughout the period under review, for both sexes and at all ages below 65 (broken down into four bands, 0–14, 15–44, 45–54, 55–64), death rates were substantially higher in Middlesbrough. The same pattern holds good for nearly all the main causes of death (Phillimore and Morris 1991). This is important, because it weighs against any explanation focused on a single cause.

If one statistic might be said to sum up the extent of the disparity between these two ostensibly similar populations, it is that mortality for the 12 years, for both sexes and all causes under the age of 65, exceeded the England and Wales average by 58 per cent in Middlesbrough, against 33 per cent in Sunderland (see Table 1). Both areas were divided into zones of higher and lesser mortality. In the pockets of highest mortality in Middlesbrough, around South Bank and Grangetown in particular, mortality under the age of 65 was over 80 per cent higher than in England and Wales; but even across relatively less severely affected parts of the selected Middlesbrough zone, local death rates still exceeded the national by around 50 per cent. This wide disparity is not a function of choosing the age of 65 as the cut-off point: indeed, as the mortality ratios in Table 1 show, the gap between the two populations is wider under 55 than in the final decade up to 65. Were death rates in the selected areas of Middlesbrough to have been at the Sunderland level, approximately 830 out of 5,300 deaths (16 per

Table 1 Premature mortality in deprived localities of Middlesbrough and Sunderland

			Middlesbrough CMR	(no. deaths)	Sunderland CMR	(no. deaths)
1975–86	Persons	0–64	158	(5301)	133	(4140)
	Men	0–64	163	(3482)	135	(2628)
	Women	0–64	149	(1819)	129	(1512)
1975–86	Persons	0–14	146	(434)	120	(298)
	Persons	15–44	145	(645)	116	(479)
	Persons	45–54	178	(1259)	138	(958)
	Persons	55–64	156	(2963)	137	(2405)
1975–77	Persons	0–64	153	(1492)	128	(1135)
1978–80	Persons	0–64	163	(1400)	133	(1081)
1981–83	Persons	0–64	156	(1243)	127	(962)
1984–86	Persons	0–64	162	(1166)	144	(962)

Note: England and Wales = 100 for each set of comparisons.
CMR = Comparative Mortality Ratio.

The CMR is equivalent to the SMR (Standardized Mortality Ratio), but based on direct instead of indirect standardization.

The two areas compared are made up of the following wards:

Middlesbrough		Sunderland
Ayresome	Beckfield	Castletown
Beechwood	Berwick Hills	Central
Church Lane	Easterside	Colliery
Grangetown	Gresham	Grindon
Grove Hill	North Ormesby	South Hylton
Pallister	Park End	Southwick
St Hilda's	South Bank	Thorney Close
Southfield	Thorntree	Town End Farm
Westbourne		

cent) of people below the age of 65 would not have occurred over the 12 years examined. To express this another way, the gap between the mortality levels of these two populations is not far short of the gap between the Sunderland and national (England and Wales) levels.

Much of the significance of this comparison stems from the scale of the contrast between two populations which have both been exposed to considerable economic hardship and insecurity. In addition, the duration of this disparity dispels any possibility that the difference between the two populations may be less 'real' than it seems. We are left, therefore, with the task of providing a sociological explanation for an unexpected differential. It is not the intention to suggest that Sunderland offers a kind of baseline for the measurement of poverty-related ill-health in northern England, from which Middlesbrough departs. Both places are equally anomalous. Nor is it the intention to suggest that the 'excess' mortality in the Teesside town is somehow independent of class and poverty, as will emerge more clearly later. For the present, it should be noted, however, that this pronounced disparity in mortality between two different working class populations is concealed in any comparison of the two entire towns. No more than an insignificant difference separated the built-up areas of Middlesbrough and Redcar (SMR 129) from the built-up area of Sunderland (SMR 121) over the period 1975–86. Whatever factors accentuate death rates in working class Middlesbrough, or mitigate them in working class Sunderland, do not appear to be operative in areas characterized by relatively greater affluence in the two towns. It is the restriction of this health differential to the poorer areas of both towns which accounts for the focus here on one section of the population in each town rather than on the whole.

Localities and local distinctiveness

With a standardized set of variables, the Census is not the obvious source to turn to if one expects to capture a sense of local peculiarity. For that, studies of specific localities are likely to be more useful, since these are at least premissed on an interest in the distinctive, indeed idiosyncratic, features of different places or local social systems. After a period of neglect, the last decade has seen waxing social scientific interest in the experience and capacities of urban localities in Britain: whether it be from a concern to depict the spatial implications of economic restructuring (Cooke 1989); to clarify the changing role of the state at the local or regional scale (Amin and Tomaney 1991; Harloe *et al.* 1990); to draw conclusions about class and social polarization in particular locales (Byrne 1989; Pahl 1984); or to bring ethnographic approaches to bear on the nature of day-to-day living in urban settings (Wallman 1984).

This work is by no means totally concerned with what makes a town or city distinctive. In any case, the microcosmic approach of an earlier generation of primarily anthropological community studies has served – perhaps unfairly – as a cautionary model, warning today's researchers of the drawbacks of a form of localism that overlooks external influences and pressures towards homogeneity, both economic and more broadly cultural (Robins 1989; Stacey 1969). Even so, the best of this work conveys a sense of the characteristics setting one place apart from another. It tends, nevertheless, to be a fairly one-sided picture, stronger on the readily observable realities – of industrial or political history, for example – than on the less readily detectable. One often looks in vain for a sense of what these outwardly observable realities add up to in people's lives, which is a point echoed in Foord *et al.* (1985:51):

> it is surprising how little is known about the impact of economic decline on individuals and communities; most of the previous studies relating economic to social change have been incomplete, focusing narrowly on just a few of the effects or on particular groups, notably the unemployed.

Yet this is where health ought to be brought into the picture, for it may suggest what life experiences add up to. Indeed, the impact of different circumstances on people's lives may only become apparent through analysis of health or mortality. I would argue that this is true of the present comparison. There have been a number of studies of Middlesbrough and Sunderland separately – most recently Middlesbrough was included in the ESRC's initiative on 'The Changing Urban and Regional System'. Beynon *et al.* (1989) refer to health, but none of the existing work on social processes (except perhaps Gladstone 1976) would lead us to anticipate that Middlesbrough offered its working class population a markedly different set of health prospects to that offered in Sunderland.

As a step towards the goal of a greater understanding of the social processes involved, I intend to chip away at three themes which I consider may be relevant to this comparison. The first revolves around the industrial environment of the two towns. The second concerns the extent to which these towns differ in their internal inequality. Finally, I shall look at the notion of lifestyle, and its possible relevance in the context of a comparison like this.

The industrial environment

Description of Middlesbrough or Sunderland generally starts with the industries which have shaped their landscapes and dominated their economies in the past 50 years and more: iron and steel and petro-chemicals on Teesside (plus shipbuilding on a lesser scale); coal-mining and shipbuilding on Wearside. The mortality sequence at the centre of this discussion, extending from 1975 to 1986, is of special interest because it spans the years of the last recession as well as the years leading into it. This was a period which saw a massive decline in employment in all four of these industries. The recession of the 1980s indeed marked the end of a long era, for by 1987 three of the four were reduced in scale to a shadow of their former importance. The sole exception was the relatively robust petro-chemicals sector, in which ICI has long been the predominant force. Indeed, it has been this industry which has set Teesside apart in the context of the north-east economy. In the last two years, shipbuilding on Wearside has ended altogether, at least for the time being. As Stubbs and Wheelock note (1986:1):

> the old image of the Wearside workforce as skilled and male simply does not fit the reality of the eighties. Not only is female employment a growing phenomenon, but the changing nature of that employment is an integral part of the industrial changes that are taking place in the locality.

The same might be said of Middlesbrough's workforce. Yet whatever the changes in industrial structure or composition of the labour force, comparison of certain features of the traditional industries is likely to be central to any attempt to explain the observed disparities in mortality. Despite severe contraction, the steel industry remains a key component of Teesside's industrial scene, while the range of petro-chemical operations in the lower Tees basin today makes it one of the largest such complexes in Europe. In Gladstone's judgement, 'it is the size of this industry that is the most striking aspect of Teesside. The concentration of large factories must be without parallel' (1976:36). All four of the heavy industries cited above carry widely recognized dangers of occupational exposure to dusts and toxic fumes. Moreover, the risks to other household members from dusts brought back into the home by workers are also being recognized. But the industries which have been the mainstay of the Teesside economy, iron and steel and petro-chemicals, have an additional, neighbourhood impact. For these operations entail exposure to air pollution which goes beyond the workforce and the workplace, to affect, in some degree, those who live in the vicinity of the plant. The distinctive impact of these industries on the Teesside environment, and the possible consequences for public health, runs like a thread through Teesside's twentieth century history. The subject of periodic speculation and enquiry, it has always been a controversial issue in local politics, with strong vested interests dampening debate (Hudson 1990). Yet because it is invariably hard to isolate any effect of air pollution from other influences bearing on the exposed population, the issue has never been resolved – one way or the other.

The Middlesbrough Locality Study refers to the fluctuations in environmental concern at various turning-points in the post-1945 development of the Tees basin, though public health implications are only touched on indirectly (see also CES 1985). Hudson, discussing the reclamation of Seal Sands at the mouth of the river for petro-chemical developments in the 1970s, summarizes an extended political and economic debate in these words (1990:73–4):

> During the mid-1960s growing concern about pollution arising from chemicals and steel production on Teesside was effectively suppressed by local politicians, many of whom had close connections with the major companies involved ... In the 1970s concern steadily grew among the local authorities, especially among some of their officers, about environmental pollution and safety hazards ... associated with land-use policies that prioritized the needs of major chemical, oil and steel developments ... Policies that encouraged polluting industries were increasingly seen as conflicting with those that sought to diversify industrial employment.

Concerns about pollution and public health may be largely absent from the economic literature, but the annual reports of the former Medical Officers of Health on Teesside provide intermittent commentary on this theme. In Sunderland, by contrast, air pollution features much less. The following remarks by the MOH in 1953 are perhaps surprisingly sanguine, but they highlight meteorological consequences of Sunderland's coastal location (Sunderland MOH Report 1953):

> The Borough of Sunderland never suffers from a pall of smoke which hangs over many industrial cities of the Midlands. This is due in great measure to the position of the Borough on the coast where there is always a free circulation of air to disturb any such accumulation.

This brief look at the industries around which the identities of both towns have been forged has two purposes: first, to draw out a palpable difference between the physical environments created by the two sets of industries, which is not just a thing of the past but continues to this day; and then to point towards the possible consequence of this environmental difference for local health patterns. The dramatic evidence on recent mortality makes it much harder than hitherto to discount the possibility of a current, and not just an historic, link between air pollution from industrial sources and health. This is a topic for future research.

It is an issue, however, which sociologists have seemed reluctant to pursue. The study of perceptions of environmental risk has been a very different matter (Bellaby 1990). Potentially influential in this regard, moreover, is recent legal interest in the possibility of making personal damage claims against local industries for causing ill-health to particular local residents as a result of pollution. Research such as this may then end up playing a part in shaping local perceptions of environmental risk. Another area of conventional sociological concern would be the breakdown of an old symbiosis between industry and neighbourhood. Hastened by the restructuring upheaval of the last decade, there has been a steady trend towards employees in these industries living outside the immediate vicinity of the works, while it appears that a declining proportion of those living close to the major plants still work there. The implications for the articulation of local opposition to industrial neighbours, and also for increased social polarization, are clear. Nevertheless, the empirical basis underpinning expressions of concern about risks to health from pollution is too easily regarded as outside the sociologist's province. All this touches on themes explored very interestingly by Benton, who summarizes the issue for sociology thus (1991:24–25):

> Environments, physical or social, may impair or enhance well-being, induce pathologies, or facilitate survival, whilst humans may act on their environments in ways which sustain or undermine the conditions of their own future survival. Sociology, surely, ought to have more to say about how these capacities are actually exercised, and with what consequences?

Given that conceptualizing the social consequences arising from the uses of technology has always been a core issue in sociology, one might have expected that the contribution of industrial pollution to the production of health differentials would attract more attention from within the discipline.

Polarization within two towns

The second topic is about the degree of social inequality manifest within each town. Might it be that Middlesbrough is a more polarized town than Sunderland? And if this were the case, would that in itself help to explain the patterns of mortality observed? To put the question another way, does Wilkinson's recent (1990) argument about the extent of social inequality and national mortality have an echo at the level of individual cities or conurbations? The evidence is not necessarily as straightforward as it seems. On the face of it, there are strong indications of greater social division in Middlesbrough than in Sunderland. Indeed, the point was made in Townsend *et al.* (1988) that Middlesbrough encompassed more pronounced social – and health – differences than anywhere else in the Northern Region. On the other hand, it could justifiably be argued that the more appropriate geographical scale for such a comparison of social inequality is the conurbation: in which case, it would be less clearcut that Teesside was vastly more unequal than Tyneside and Wearside together (although the dramatically high mortality in working class areas does make it more unequal in health).

The extent to which housing areas are segregated on class lines provides the most concrete symbol of urban inequality. In many places, it is the so-called 'outer estates' – not always as peripheral as they were at the time of construction – which represent the extremity of local deprivation. Byrne has suggested (personal communication) that in Middlesbrough the post-1945 rehousing programme 'remade' the town on a scale which had few parallels outside Glasgow, resulting in an extremely high proportion of the population living in outer estates. Certainly, the Max Lock Plan of 1946 laid the basis for an enormous programme of building that lasted into the 1970s, with the estates making up the single tract of East Middlesbrough forming the largest component. On any of the conventional indicators, these are areas of substantial deprivation (CES 1984, 1985; Townsend *et al.* 1988). It is not clear, however, that Middlesbrough was 'remade' on a drastically different scale than Sunderland. According to CES (1984:2), the number of people living in outer estates defined as deprived in both towns were almost identical (in 1971); although these numbers do account for a higher proportion of the total population in Middlesbrough. Statistics in Dennis' study (1970) of Sunderland's housing programme also tend to reinforce an impression of the similarity of the two towns.

Yet these bald figures are only a small part of the picture. The more elusive comparative task is to look at the way that housing policies have been framed and implemented; at the quality of the housing; and at the provision of services and facilities within each of these estates. Issues here include the phase of post-war rebuilding, and, linked to this, political and policy shifts in assumptions about the people for whom different estates were designed. Resolving comparative questions of this kind is beyond the scope of this contribution, and may be altogether too ambitious. But a couple of observations point towards the possibility of qualitatively greater dislocation in people's lives, in working class Middlesbrough, as rehousing plans were executed. First, primary health care provision has been much more dispersed in Sunderland, with health centres closer to patients' homes. By contrast, in Middlesbrough, centralizing primary care in the town's Cleveland Centre has resulted in long journeys for the majority. It appears, also, that roads present more of a danger to pedestrians, particularly children, in the poorer areas of Middlesbrough, judging by the fact that children's mortality from road traffic accidents is over three times higher than in the comparable areas of Sunderland (Phillimore and Morris 1991). Numbers may be small, but this is a staggering divergence between the two places, strongly suggesting that the outer estates of Sunderland are laid out in ways that are more sensitive to the needs of daily activity.

A separate theme concerns the relations of class to which the characteristic industries of these towns give rise. On the Registrar-General's model of class, over 80 per cent of households were categorized as having a manual 'head' in both areas in 1981. In Middlesbrough, however, the proportion of semi-skilled and unskilled households was higher than in Sunderland (44 per cent against 34 per cent of all households) (Phillimore and Morris 1991). The sociologically interesting question is how much this difference reflects a 'real' divergence in class experience, and how much it is merely a by-product of OPCS coding conventions. Deprivation measures, it should be remembered, came into fashion partly as a result of misgivings about what it was that occupational class actually described. In this comparison, there are grounds for suggesting that the Registrar-General's model may reflect a potentially significant difference not discernible in conventional measures of deprivation. Admittedly, this difference is created on the basis largely of male occupations: but in fact there is little evidence of divergence in female employment patterns in the two populations, with similar types of occupation and proportions of part-time to full-time female employment. On the other hand, one difference between the four heavy industries may have indirect repercussions for health patterns. Shipbuilding and coal mining have tended to give comparatively greater autonomy and control to the workforce than steel and chemical production. This is a separate matter from skill, of craft predominance in the shipyards against process work in steel and chemicals. In any case, to classify process workers generically as semi-skilled is rudimentary in the extreme. The point to make is simply that relative autonomy and control at work may be one facet of hidden differences in class culture between the two places. This leads to my final topic.

Fears, values, habits – and lifestyle

In looking first at the impact of certain heavy industries on the health of the surrounding population, and then at the physical manifestations of polarization and inequality within cities, I have biased the discussion towards those structures which shape and constrain people's lives. But what of human agency? Are there perhaps differences in the ways in which people themselves shape their environments in these two towns, which may contribute to the mortality differences?

In relation to health issues, this is the domain of 'lifestyle'. I recognize that, outside the field of health, lifestyle has its theorists (above all Bourdieu 1984:169–225), who are intrigued by its semiotic role in defining power relations. The link between lifestyle and capitalism's propensity to define new commodities, and the restless displacement of one cultural token by another, also seem to exert a fascination for some commentators trying to define a supposedly post-modern condition. But these preoccupations scarcely impinge on the conceptualization and use of lifestyle in a health context. Instead, the existence and defining characteristics of lifestyles are taken for granted. A double reduction takes place. The role of human agency in the reproduction of social life and culture is reduced to lifestyle; and lifestyle is then conventionally limited to four habits, selected for their known influence upon health and their amenability to rudimentary measurement. I refer of course to smoking, eating, drinking and physical exercise (Cox *et al.* 1987). The difficulty with lifestyle so construed lies not with the separate elements – no researcher into health would ignore the significance of smoking, for example. It lies with the reluctance to bring to bear on health a more complex understanding of how people act as they do. In place of a vision of how social activity and the decisions we make reproduce the structures which in turn constrain us, we resort to a concept – lifestyle – with inescapable connotations of the idioms of 'consumer choice' and 'individual responsibility'. No amount of stressing that lifestyles are socially constructed and not simply freely chosen evades the individualism of the concept.

Frustration at the unsatisfactoriness of the notion of lifestyle is increased by its ubiquity and contemporary influence. Yet there exist other lenses through which to look at the very features of life so distorted when viewed simply as lifestyle. Part of the interest of a comparison between the selected localities of Middlesbrough and Sunderland is that another lens is definitely required. It seems implausible to imagine that these two working class populations, living scarcely 25 miles apart, eat, drink, smoke and exercise in a different fashion. But this is a rather superficial level of resemblance. Are there perhaps other conventions, habits and forms of behaviour through which deeper differences may be apparent? For example, in the last section, I touched on the question of control and autonomy people have in their lives, and the implications this might have for day-to-day experience.

One of the alternative lenses available is the concept of the moral economy. This concept needs some clarification, as different shades of meaning and emphasis have been given to it by different writers (see Parry and Bloch 1989 for a valuable discussion). But in the present context, Scott points the way when he states (1976:2):

> If the Great Depression left an indelible mark on the fears, values, and habits of a whole generation of Americans, can we imagine the impact of periodic food crises on the fears, values, and habits of rice farmers in monsoon Asia?

The emphasis on fears, values and habits is the crux of the matter, while the reference to the Great Depression serves as a useful reminder that the concept of the moral economy has utility in market just as much as non-market milieux. Scott – and others writing from a similar perspective (for example, Greenough 1980) – make us conceptualize daily routines, decision-making and choice against a background of a struggle to survive. Just as important, the struggle to get by has inseparable physical, practical and moral dimensions. Poverty – and in Greenough's moving study, sheer famine – are thus approached, not by way of statistical indicators, but through insight into how people act in difficult circumstances. In Greenough's words: 'What, in detail, do Indian peasants do when famine looms ... *within* the peasant household, where distinctions begin to be made between those who are more and those who are less deserving of survival' (1980:205, 208). The scale may be less catastrophic, but this is exactly the task that confronts us in trying to account for health differences of the kind under discussion in this chapter.

All this reminds us is that there exist other, more socially grounded, traditions of writing about personal choice and responsibility or individual decisions about consumption. I have drawn attention to one which has had a lot to say, moreover, about extremes of poverty and ill-health. If it is one which emphasizes that 'choice' is generally a misnomer for 'compromise' or 'necessity' where resources are few, that is simply to echo Graham's depiction of the inner rationale of coping strategies in poorer households, summed up in the words 'health choices are more accurately seen as health compromises' (1984:187). In short, much remains to be learned about how to conceptualize the ways that people's decisions may influence their health.

Conclusion

This is not an analysis which lends itself to sharp conclusions. The three themes I have discussed focus attention on a diverse set of possible influences on health. Yet if we are to clarify how different kinds of life experience combine to produce differing health outcomes, then we must find ways of encompassing such diversity. In this comparative case-study of historical processes at work in two neighbouring towns, each theme seems to me to require closer scrutiny, going well beyond the kind of correlational analysis of existing data sets that has defined the limits of so much work on health inequalities.

An axiom of sociological interest in health inequalities has been that levels of health provide a sensitive guide to the conditions in which people's lives are led. We should not overstate the case. Not everything that distinguishes one social milieu from another, for example, will show up in the health record, and it would be mechanistic in the extreme to suggest that what is sociologically significant is necessarily significant for health. Nonetheless, levels of mortality summarize the cumulative impact of multiple influences upon people's lives, in a way that has no parallel among routine socio-economic indicators (Wilkinson 1986:2–3). Moreover, to turn the proposition around, where marked disparities in health are observed between populations or places, there must be a strong presumption of significant underlying differences in the circumstances and conditions of people's lives. Whatever census indicators may suggest about the broad socio-economic similarity of these two populations in Middlesbrough and Sunderland, there must also be certain striking differences in the lives people lead in these towns in order to have produced such dissimilar mortality experience. The task here has been to explore what some of these differences might be. This is as much about identifying comparatively favourable influences in Sunderland as it is about damaging influences in Middlesbrough. To the extent that Sunderland's achievement is a product of relatively recent policy, and not just a legacy of history or an accident of geography, it offers some kind of model in the context of levels of mortality in the Northern Region. In Tyneside during the early 1980s, for instance, similarly deprived areas experienced mortality under the age of 65 mid-way between Sunderland and Middlesbrough levels (an aggregate SMR of 143 for 23 Tyneside wards in 1981–83). This chapter is a reminder, therefore, that the characteristics of places may be as important as the characteristics of people for an understanding of particular patterns of health – all the more so when the latter is narrowly conceived.

Acknowledgements

In writing this paper I have benefitted greatly from discussion with David Byrne and George Courtice.

References

Amin, A. and Tomaney, J. (1991), 'Illusions of prosperity: the political economy of urban and regional regeneration in north east England', in Fasenfest, P. and Meyer, P. (eds), *The Politics of Local Economic Policy Formation*, London: Macmillan.

Bellaby, P. (1990), 'To risk or not to risk? Uses and limitations of Mary Douglas on risk-acceptability for understanding health and safety at work and road accidents', *Sociological Review*, **38**:465–83.

Benton, T. (1991), 'Biology and social science: why the return of the repressed should be given a (cautious) welcome', *Sociology*, **25**:1–29.

Beynon, H., Hudson, R., Lewis, J., Sadler, D. and Townsend, A. (1989), '"It's all falling apart here": coming to terms with the future in Teesside', in Cooke, P. (ed.), *Localities: the Changing Face of Urban Britain*, London: Unwin Hyman.

Bourdieu, P. (1984), *Distinction: a Social Critique of the Judgement of Taste*, London: Routledge and Kegan Paul.

Byrne, D. (1989), *Beyond the Inner City*, Milton Keynes: Open University Press.

Carstairs, V. and Morris, R. (1989), 'Deprivation and mortality: an alternative to social class?', *Community Medicine*, **11**:210–19.

Centre for Environmental Studies (1984), *Outer Estates in Britain: Preliminary Comparison of Four Outer Estates*, CES Paper 23, London: CES.

Centre for Environmental Studies (1985), *Outer Estates in Britain: East Middlesbrough Case Study*, CES Paper 26, London: CES.

Congdon, P. (1988), 'Deprivation in London wards: mortality and unemployment trends in the 1980's', *The Statistician*, **37**:451–72.

Cooke, P. (ed.) (1989), *Localities: the Changing Face of Urban Britain*, London: Unwin Hyman.

Cox, B., Blaxter, M., Buckle, A. *et al.* (1987), *The Health and Lifestyle Survey*, London: Health Promotion Research Trust.

Dennis, N. (1970), *People and Planning: the Sociology of Housing in Sunderland*, London: Faber and Faber.
DHSS (1980), Inequalities in Health: Report of a Research Working Group, *The Black Report*, London: HMSO.
Foord, J., Robinson, F. and Sadler, D. (1985), *The Quiet Revolution: Social and Economic Change on Teesside, 1965–85*, Newcastle: BBC (NE).
Gladstone, F. (1976), *The Politics of Planning*, London: Temple Smith.
Graham, H. (1984), *Women, Health and the Family*, Brighton: Wheatsheaf.
Greenough, P. (1980), 'Indian famines and peasant victims: the case of Bengal in 1943–44', *Modern Asian Studies*, **14**:205–35.
Harloe, M., Pickvance, C. and Urry, J. (eds) (1990), *Place, Policy and Politics: Do Localities Matter?*, London: Unwin Hyman.
Hudson, R. (1990), 'Trying to revive an infant Hercules: the rise and fall of local authority modernization policies on Teesside', in Harloe, M., Pickvance, C. and Urry, J. (eds), *Place, Policy and Politics: Do Localities Matter?*, London: Unwin Hyman.
Pahl, R. (1984), *Divisions of Labour*, Oxford: Basil Blackwell.
Parry, J. and Bloch, M. (eds) (1989), *Money and the Morality of Exchange*, Cambridge: Cambridge University Press.
Phillimore, P. (1990), 'Mortality variations within two poor areas in North-East England', *The Statistician*, **39**:373–83.
Phillimore, P. and Morris, D. (1991), 'Discrepant legacies: premature mortality in two industrial towns', *Social Science and Medicine*, **33**, (2):139–152.
Robins, K. (1989), Global Times, *Marxism Today*, (Dec.).
Scott, J. (1976), *The Moral Economy of the Peasant: Rebellion and Subsistence in Southeast Asia*, New Haven: Yale University Press.
Stacey, M. (1969), 'The myth of community studies', *British Journal of Sociology*, **20**:134–45.
Stubbs, C. and Wheelock, J. (1986), 'Women's work: gender and the Wearside local economy', Sunderland Polytechnic.
Sunderland Medical Officer of Health (1953), Annual Report Sunderland County Borough.
Townsend, P. and Davidson, N. (1982), *Inequalities in Health: the Black Report*, Harmondsworth: Penguin.
Townsend, P., Corrigan, P. and Kowarzik, U. (1987), *Poverty and Labour in London: a Survey of Londoners' Living Standards*, London: Low Pay Unit.
Townsend, P., Phillimore, P. and Beattie, A. (1988), *Health and Deprivation: Inequality and the North*, London: Croom Helm.
Wallman, S. (1984), *Eight London Households*, London: Tavistock.
Wilkinson, R. (ed.) (1986), *Class and Health: Research and Longitudinal Data*, London: Tavistock.
Wilkinson, R. (1990), 'Income distribution and mortality: a "natural" experiment', *Sociology of Health and Illness*, **12**:4, 391.

10 The health costs of Britain's industrialization: A perspective from the Celtic periphery

Rory Williams

Did the health and prosperity of the British population improve or decline in the course of the industrial revolution? The fall in national mortality which accompanied and followed the industrial revolution during most of the nineteenth century is perhaps the greatest single landmark in the modern medical landscape; and it has lent a powerful argument to the optimists in the debate.

There are, however, strong health arguments in the pessimists' camp as well; and the present chapter arises out of puzzlement about one notorious instance. It looks at the regional health experience of contemporary and historical Clydeside, and attempts an initial exploration of one factor which might account for that experience, and which might predict similar health experiences elsewhere. This factor is the major part played in Clydeside's industrialization by immigrants from the Scottish Highlands and from Ireland. This chapter is in no sense a completed survey, but a flying column sent to find out the limits of a large and only partially charted terrain. Reference is made later to hypotheses which will carry the inquiry further.

The issues involved in the controversy about industrialization have been summarized elsewhere (Floud *et al.* 1990; Cage 1987; Taylor 1975). The contention is between three broad schools of thought, or more accurately, perhaps three broad coalitions, each appealing to a certain range of explanatory models. First is the neoclassical school, perhaps the most unified, which argues that production rose faster than population, both in agriculture and industry, and that market forces were sufficiently well developed to distribute the benefits to the mass of the increasing population in rising real wages and reduced mortality.

Second comes a coalition of some of the more pessimistic economists together with the more optimistic egalitarians and radicals, suggesting that while there certainly was unprecedented and sustained growth per capita, there were also very much increased inequalities, with the rich gaining enormously and the poor little or not at all. According to the explanation preferred, either landowners or capitalists (or both) cornered the benefits, and they did it variously because the increasing demand for food, or the use of enclosure or eviction, favoured the landlords, or because price inflation, or capital-intensive innovation or monopolistic collusion in holding down wages, or the weak bargaining power of labour, favoured the employer.

Finally, there is what may be called the catastrophic school, comprising various sorts of Malthusian, together with the bleakest interpreters of increasing inequalities, who agree that for a very substantial part, even for a majority, of the population, things got worse. This was because food resources, or industrial resources, were insufficient to sustain the rising population, or at least to sustain it while landlords or capitalists cornered benefits through the processes already listed, especially if the wealth they cornered was not distributed or used to produce or employ.

Quantitative measures for the investigation of these questions have fallen into three broad categories. First come indices of real wages, and for convenience we may include with these the studies of food consumption and of the supply of housing, fuel and clothing, together with computations based on national income per capita. Secondly, and more broadly, appeal has been made to the evidence that country people migrated in such large numbers, and for so long a period to the towns. Finally, reference is often made to measures of health. The astonishing fall in the death rate during the nineteenth century, outstripping all effects of age composition and age-specific rates, was an obvious topic, and it was soon argued that economic factors might explain this rather better than medical factors. In what follows, while there is some discussion of the issues concerning real income and migration, the chief emphasis is on those concerning health.

Sources of optimism – the national evidence

The problem of this chapter begins from the conflict between national evidence and, initially, the evidence from Clydeside. The national evidence on real wages is nearly all English, with a distinct bias to the south. Figure 1 gives a typical curve for the eighteenth and nineteenth centuries, in which the most serious dip is during the high prices of the Napoleonic Wars. Otherwise, while there is some evidence of decline in the second half of the eighteenth century, the general trend is firmly upward, including the period from 1815 to 1870 when the great growth of industrial cities took place. The most important regional exception to the picture unearthed so far, excluding Clydeside (which is discussed shortly), is the series for Lanca-

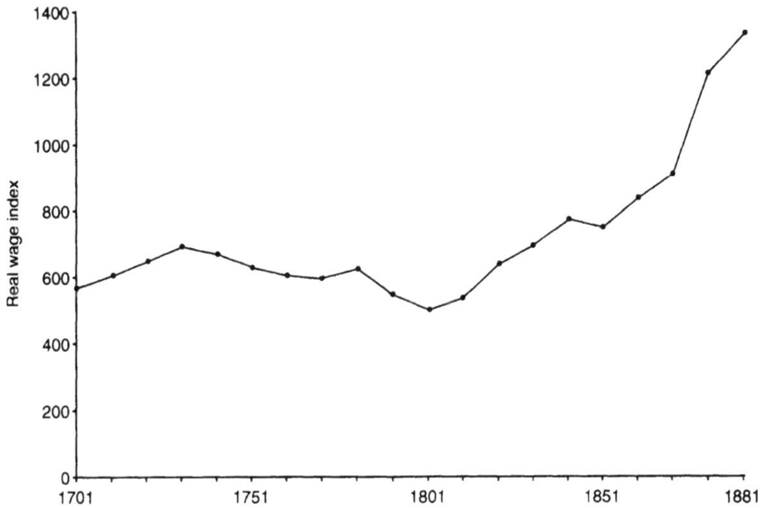

Source: Wrigley and Schofield.

Figure 1 Real wages, England 1701–1881

shire up to 1800, which reveals growth throughout the eighteenth century (Gilboy 1975).

This optimistic picture is corroborated by the picture for migration to the towns, if one accepts that migration expressed a genuine preference. The British Isles, alone in Western Europe, experienced a continuous growth in the urban proportion of the population between 1500 and 1800 (de Vries 1984:39), and by the time that good migration indices were available for England and Wales, after 1851, the flood of population moving from rural counties to the industrial centres dominated and indeed obliterated all other tendencies (Friedlander and Roshier 1966a).

Finally, the trends in national death rates are in the same direction (Figure 2). During the period of national registration, the trends in the crude death rate in England and Wales and in Scotland are both downward, indeed spectacularly so between 1870 and 1920. There is a hint of an upward movement in the initial years of both series, but the careful work done in England by back projection techniques on parish records before the

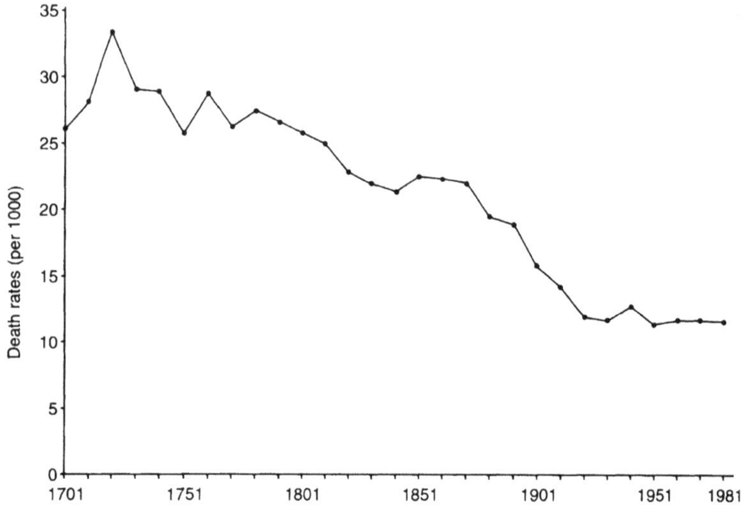

Source: Wrigley and Schofield, RG.

Figure 2 Crude death rates, England 1701–1981

period of registration suggests that there is little significance in this (Wrigley and Schofield 1981). Rather the trend, after the fluctuating mortality of the early eighteenth century settles down, is more or less continuously downward, with at most a pause, or a moment of slight fluctuation both down and up, between 1820 and 1860. Similarly in Scotland, the death rates retrievable for the middle and end of the eighteenth century suggest, albeit at rather wide intervals, a parallel downward trend (Flinn 1977). There is, then, a broad harmony in these overall measures, which would lead us to conclude that the growth of industrial employment and industrial cities supervened smoothly on the trend, already apparent, to improvement in the market and the distribution system in the eighteenth century. Industrialism and the market continued to grow in symbiosis, and the result, it would seem, was in all these respects beneficial. It is against this picture that the equivalent data for Clydeside comes as such a shock.

The problem of Clydeside

There is no index of real wages available for Clydeside through the whole of the nineteenth century. An index has been constructed for the period from 1810 to 1840, with a gap between 1819 and 1836 (Cage 1983), and there are data on food prices, rent and wages in varying occupations at varying intervals thereafter (Slaven 1975:154–9). None of this can give a very firm picture, but certain outlines are apparent which do not conform to the national trends just described.

First, the falling prices after the Napoleonic War did not, as elsewhere, tend to a rise in real wages. On the contrary, what evidence there is suggests a fall which was continued, with minor fluctuations, through to 1840; and in the 1840s themselves, unemployment and hardship were notoriously severe. Such recovery as took place in the 1850s was interrupted by the crash of 1856/7, and it is only by 1870 that we find evidence of skilled occupations definitely exceeding the standard of living prevalent towards the end of the Napoleonic War, while more populous but less skilled occupations such as spinning are only just approaching that level again. There could not be a more striking contrast with the English figures shown earlier, where the end of the Napoleonic War represented not a standard to be recovered, but a nadir from which real wages leapt up ebulliently and pretty well continuously thereafter.

Studies of the consumption of goods on Clydeside during this period are at present feasible only for housing, but this confirms and strengthens the impression. Figures for persons per room are available in the Scottish Census from 1861 onwards, and before that it is possible, with great caution, to estimate them from the figures for persons per house from 1801. The caution is necessary because definitions of a house, in cities of tenement flats, proved extraordinarily problematic, not least because in mid-century the organizers of the Scottish Census had to struggle with inappropriate definitions imposed on them from England. This makes the figures of persons per house unusable from 1851–71; but even before this, it is demonstrable that the Edinburgh enumerators recorded the whole tenement as a house, while the Glasgow enumerators recorded each individual flat as a house. However both cities, after apparently trying to switch definitions in 1811, seem to have settled down to their own consistent practice up to 1841. From this, there can be little doubt that in the first half of the century, the level of overcrowding in Glasgow was rapidly increasing (Figure 3). When the figures for persons per room become available, the crowding seems still to be at its worst, but from a high point in 1871 it falls steadily thereafter. Thus in the largest single item of consumption available to them, Glaswegians became conspicuously and steadily poorer throughout the years of industrial take-off up to 1870.

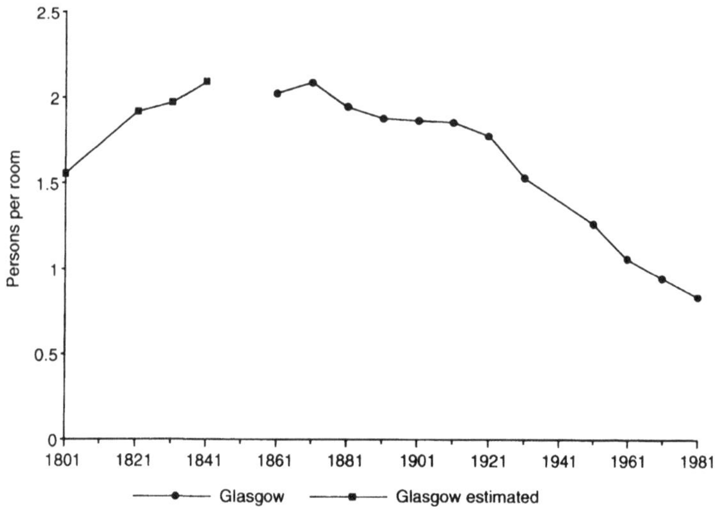

Source: Census.

Figure 3 Glasgow: Persons per room

Yet for all that, a great flood of migrants were coming into Clydeside from the countryside throughout these years. Were they then convinced that they would better their way of life by so doing? A certain caution is induced when more particular inquiry is made about where these migrants were coming from. Of the vast population which had immigrated into West Scotland by the mid-century, nearly two thirds came from Ireland or the Highlands (Slaven 1975:143). These are years when in many parts of the Highlands, evictions and relocations were taking place to make room for sheep and deer forests. And in Ireland an inextricable tangle of agrarian problems was helping to bring the Irish rural economy to a state of extreme fragility. In both areas, finally, the population was increasing rapidly, and the part of it which held on was forced more and more to rely on the potato for survival; and in both, therefore, the arrival of the potato blight in the 1840s had catastrophic consequences. Thus we should be wary about taking the consequent migrations to be an expression of preferences for the urban industrial way of life.

Of all indices of industrial welfare, however, the death rate is, in the case of Glasgow, the best attested. Exceptionally careful death records were maintained there from 1783 on, and this permits a reasonably reliable rate to be obtained at the census of population taken for the First Statistical Account 1791 (Sinclair 1795), as well as at subsequent local censuses by age and sex, conducted from 1821 until the Registrar General took over (Flinn 1977). Figure 4 shows that from a relatively high figure in the 1790s, not untypical of cities in the eighteenth century, in comparison with the national death rate, Glasgow had succeeded by 1821, in bringing down the rate to within a point or two of the English national figure. Such levels of health were not to be seen again in the city for more than sixty years. As industrial output rose and the great surge of immigration began, death rates spiralled upwards to an appalling peak around 1851 and continued at the levels of the crisis years of the early eighteenth century in England, until after 1871. These are crude death rates, but age standardization would only

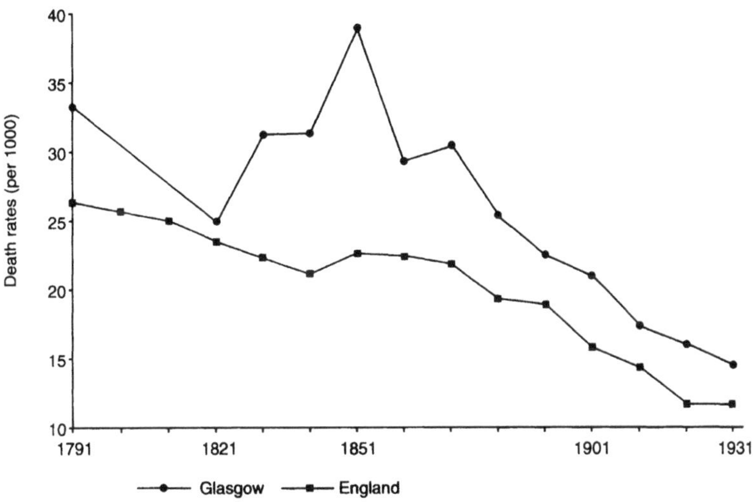

Source: Flinn *et al.* (Glasgow).

Figure 4 Crude death rates, Glasgow vs England 1791–1931

increase the effect, since Glasgow had smaller proportions in the vulnerable age groups.[1]

Nor was this all; for the fall in the death rate that began thereafter was never able to do more than run parallel with the English fall, taking a similar curve, but starting at a much higher point on the graph; and it remains above the English curve today as it was towards the end of the nineteenth century. Thus the relative position of Glasgow today would seem to have been fixed by the experience of the mid-nineteenth century, a fact which raises important questions about the factors which could be responsible for maintaining this kind of continuity.

This evidence thus forces upon us the question, was Clydeside a grotesque exception to the national picture of beneficent industrialization? Or was it merely a rather better-recorded example of conditions which prevailed in a number of places? And if the latter, how can we diagnose and distinguish those places which emulated Clydeside's experience, from those that followed the pattern of, say, the south of England? And what is the relation between these two nations within the nation?

Theoretical predictors of the Clydeside syndrome

It is already apparent that Clydeside had at least two distinctive formative characteristics – its industrial base in heavy manufacturing, and its recruiting grounds in Ireland and the Highlands. In the search for theoretical parallels, the second characteristic – relating Clydeside to the kind of culture and economy found to the north and west – is the more neglected in studies of industrialism, and needs the more careful exposition. That done, I consider some of the links between these recruiting grounds and other industrial centres in Britain. And finally, I review theoretical accounts of these links, and draw out hypotheses relating to health.

The economic sector represented by Ireland and the Highlands Ireland and the Scottish Highlands belonged, in the early nineteenth century, to a region of the British Isles characterized by the agriculture of smallholders, holding tenancies of very variable security, payable in cash, kind, or labour, with a wide spectrum of activities which often included herding or fishing, carried out for the most part by family members, and broadly aimed at subsistence as the first priority, though often with an element of cash cropping alongside. They were, in other words, dominated by a peasant mode of production (Shanin 1990), at least as far as the lifetime experience of the mass of the population went – the aspect of the economy which is most relevant to the reasons for population change and emigration. From the point of view of commercial production and export, of course, they looked quite different, and both the Highlands and, in particular, Ireland also had an advanced export agriculture, based on large farms or pastures, commercial specialization and hired labour. But this did not overturn the peasant basis of common life; indeed the two modes of production often lived in symbiosis.

The way in which a peasant mode of production can co-exist, to mutual advantage, with capitalist agriculture, the peasant mode dominating popular experience even as the capitalist mode dominates commerce, is well illustrated by Ian Carter's portrayal of another part of this peasant region – the Scottish north-east (Carter 1979). Here, throughout the century, the peasant mode supplied skilled young recruits for the capitalist mode as the children grew up, and retrieved them as men when the opportunity to inherit or solicit small tenancies became available in middle life. For this reason, hired labour was marginally more numerous than family labour on north-east farms throughout the century, and to that extent, it is capitalist agriculture which seems marginally to have dominated; yet when we look at lifetime chances, because capitalist agriculture ran largely on adolescent labour, those who stayed on the land still spent most of their lives in peasant smallholdings – grew up on them, and took tenancies on them from their mid-years onward. Thus, the peasant ethos remained stronger than the capitalist ethos in popular experience.

How can we identify those areas of the British Isles in which a peasant majority still counterbalanced a commercially more productive capitalist minority in the early nineteenth century? In the light of Ian Carter's study, a key indication would seem to be the lifetime chances of hired labour becoming farmers in their own right, and this can be approximated by looking at the ratio of farmers to hired labourers in different areas. In the north-east of Scotland in 1851, the number of male farmers was 50 per cent of the number of male agricultural labourers and farm servants, suggesting that, after allowing for some attrition among the latter due to mortality, migration or later change of occupation, a tenancy was still a prospect for most of these (mainly young) men to look forward to.

If this was so in north-east Scotland, we would expect farmers to be in even more favourable ratio to farm workers in Ireland and the Highlands. In Ireland, the proportion of large farms was even smaller than in north-east Scotland, where farms of over 100 acres were, even in 1885, no more than a sixth of all holdings (Carter 1979:29; Mokyr 1983:19). And everywhere in Ireland, a sector characterized by subsistence and barter undergirded the export economy (Mokyr 1983:20–4).

There are unfortunately considerable problems about the 1851 Census definition of 'farmers' and 'labourers' in Ireland and the Scottish Highlands (see Appendix). But if we estimate all male occupiers of over an acre of land in Ireland in 1851, the ratio of these landholders to male labour stands at 79 per cent. The ratio was probably a little lower before the famine, for while occupiers holding small acreages shrank disproportionately between 1841 and 1851, true labourers with less than an acre shrank most of all; but this ratio of landholders to labour must nevertheless, like the analogous ratio of farmers to labour, have risen steadily for the rest of the century (Fitzpatrick 1980). Paradoxically, the famine and the emigration merely confirmed Ireland as a peasant economy, the tendency being especially marked in Ulster and Connaught, but remaining strong by British standards even in Munster and Leinster.

In the Scottish Highlands, meanwhile, a similar reconstruction reveals that in 1851 the number of male farmers (including crofters) stood at 72 per cent of the number of male labourers – a result very similar to that for

Table 1 Census of Great Britain and Ireland 1851 (males): Farmers per 100 agricultural labourers and farm servants, by region

Region	Farmers per 100 agricultural labourers and farm servants
Ireland (see Appendix)	79
Wales with Monmouthshire	68
Scotland	
Highlands	72
North-east	50
North-central	33
South-west	31
South-east	15
England	
Northern	43
North-west	49
Yorkshire	49
North Midlands	30
South-west	28
West Midlands	24
South Midlands	14
Eastern counties	15
South-east counties	13

Source: Census 1851 vol. 2 pp. ccxliv, 915f. Scottish counties assigned as follows: *Highlands* – Orkney and Shetland, Caithness, Sutherland, Ross and Cromarty, Inverness, Argyll, Bute; *North-east* – Aberdeen, Banff, Elgin, Nairn; *North-central* – Kincardine, Forfar, Perth, Stirling; *South-west* – Dumbarton, Renfrew, Lanark, Ayr, Kirkcudbright, Dumfries, Wigtown; *South-east* – Fife, Kinross, Clackmannan, Linlithgow, Edinburgh, Haddington, Peebles, Selkirk, Roxburgh, Berwick. Figures for Orkney and Shetland, Sutherland, Inverness and Argyll corrected for misallocation of crofters to agricultural labourers in 1851 (see Appendix).

Ireland. These figures for Ireland and the Highlands can now be compared with those for the rest of Britain in 1851 (Table 1). The closest resemblance is obviously with Wales, where again smallholding tenants were more numerous than elsewhere in Britain, and farmers' sons again often worked for neighbouring farmers for a period when they grew up, living in with the family (Howell 1977). The similar arrangements in north-east Scotland have already been noted. On the other hand, Alan Macfarlane has argued that England never had a peasantry (Macfarlane 1978). We should be cautious of assuming this of the upland areas of the Pennines, Cumbria and Northumbria, for here smallholding with live-in labour was also a feature (Chambers and Mingay 1966:19,95; Howell 1977:94; Macfarlane 1978:71f., 91; Clapham 1926:110–13), and the ratio of farmers to labourers was relatively high in 1851. But south or east of all these regions were marginal areas – in North-central and South-west Scotland, in the North and West Midlands and South-west of England – where the ratio was lower; and in two large zones – roughly south of the Wash and east of the Cotswolds in England, and south of the Tay and Ochils and east of the Clyde basin in Scotland, large capitalist farms confronted landless labourers with very little chance of gaining a holding themselves.

There were thus two broad sectors in the early nineteenth-century agriculture of the British Isles, with margins of intermediate farming practices between them; and it is a striking fact that the proportions of the population found within each of these sectors then were very different from the proportions we are accustomed to today. In 1821, when the census covered all the British Isles for the first time, out of a total population of 21 million, 38 per cent lived in the classic areas of peasant dominance in Ireland, the Scottish Highlands, and Wales, with a further substantial proportion in the Scottish north-east and the English Lakes and Dales; while only 23 per cent lived in the classic areas of agricultural capitalism (Census of Great Britain 1821:xxxii–xxxv; Vaughan and Fitzpatrick 1978:3). In short, the agricultural capitalism of the south-east of England and Scotland, hitherto so thoroughly documented, was peripheral in popular experience, and the peasant agriculture of the north and west of the British Isles was at the core of that experience. But all this was about to change.

The link of the peasant sector with the industrial centres It was the peasant populations of the British Isles that collapsed as industrialism gained ground. While the south-eastern areas of England and Scotland maintained their proportion of the islands' population into the twentieth century, the growth of the industrial cities coincided with a headlong decline in the proportion of the population living in the peasant areas of the first half of the century. Not only did these areas not sustain the population growth that occurred in the areas of agricultural capitalism, but their absolute numbers actually shrank away as well. In Ireland, the greatest single part of the patchwork, the population fell from 6.8 million in 1821 (32 per cent of the population of the British Isles, and by no means yet at Ireland's peak) to 4.4 million in 1911 (by then less than 10 per cent). And in rural Wales, and to a lesser extent the Highlands, numbers also plummetted not only relatively but absolutely (Census of Great Britain 1821:xxxii–xxxv; Census of England and Wales 1911, vol. 1:3f.; Census of Scotland 1911, vol. 2:xxiv; Vaughan and Fitzpatrick 1978:3; Hechter 1975:187; Flinn 1977:306).

These figures thus underline the fact that the industrial transformation was also, and perhaps primarily, a colossal transformation in the areas where peasant modes of production had held sway. Certainly there were also, by 1861, substantial movements out of the homelands of agricultural capitalism – out of south and east England towards London, and out of the Borders of Scotland, probably mainly towards Glasgow and Edinburgh. But London and Edinburgh were not the centres of industrialization – rather, they were commercial and service cities which were benefiting from the already long-entrenched development of the market, rather than from industrial manufacture as such. Compared with the catchment areas for these cities, the source populations in peasant areas were not only larger, but they also provided some of the highest net rates of emigrants per head (Friedlander and Roshier 1966b:Table III.5; Vaughan and Fitzpatrick 1978:261; O'Grada 1975 and 1978; Flinn 1977:464–5).

Were these peasant areas characteristic sources for the specifically industrial cities? Since Ireland was the largest single source area of this type, an indication of the answer to this question can be gained by looking at those cities in Britain where the proportion of Irish-born adults was already over 10 per cent by 1851. The list includes Liverpool, Manchester and Stockport in the future north-western conurbations, Newcastle and Gateshead in the Tyneside conurbation, Bradford in the West Yorkshire conurbation, Newport in Monmouthshire, and Glasgow, Paisley, Kilmarnock and Dundee in the Scottish central belt (Table 2). Inclusion of the Welsh emigration would, of course, reinforce the link with other industrial centres in South Wales, and inclusion of the Highland emigration would further reinforce the link with the Scottish central belt. Similarly, emigration from the Lakes and Dales further fuelled industry in Lancashire and Yorkshire (Redford 1976:183). Meanwhile, if the proportion of Irish is lowered to 5 per cent, virtually none of the greatest 20–30 industrial cities is left out, barring Sheffield and Nottingham and one or two others, while of the remaining 30–40 largely commercial and administrative centres among the chief cities of Britain, very few have such proportions of Irish. Thus there is a *prima facie* case for investigating whether there is not an important connection between industrialism and the breaking of the peasant mode of production in Ireland, northern Scotland, Wales and possibly northern England.

Table 2 Census of Great Britain 1851: Percentage born in Ireland of adult population (age 20+) in principal towns (south to north)

1 Over 20%	**%**	**4 Other principal towns**
Liverpool	29	Truro
Glasgow	23	Plymouth
Dundee	22	Exeter
		Dorchester
2 10–20%		Bristol
		Bath
Newport (Monmouthshire)	14	Salisbury
Wolverhampton	10	Southampton
Stockport	12	Brighton
Manchester and Salford	17	Canterbury
Bradford	11	Maidstone
Carlisle	11	Reading
Gateshead	11	Oxford
Newcastle upon Tyne	10	Gloucester
Dumfries	10	Worcester
Kilmarnock	17	Shrewsbury
Paisley	17	Dudley
		Coventry
3 5–9%		Northampton
		Bedford
Portsmouth	5	Cambridge
Winchester	8	Colchester
London	6	Ipswich
Swansea	6	Yarmouth
Merthyr Tydfil	7	Norwich
Birmingham	6	Bury St Edmonds
Chester	9	Leicester
Macclesfield	8	Boston
Bolton	9	Lincoln
Preston	9	Nottingham
Leeds	6	Derby
Halifax	7	Hull
Huddersfield	7	Sheffield
York	6	Lancaster
Durham	8	South Shields
Sunderland	7	Perth
Tynemouth	5	Aberdeen
Edinburgh and Leith	8	Inverness

Theoretical formulations of the link The nature of this connection between the peasant areas and the industrial cities can be interpreted in very different ways. In what follows, I summarize three well-known types of interpretation, and at the same time I consider whether they offer any clues, not only to the standard of living of the emigrants before and after migration and to their reasons for migrating, but also to patterns of health experience like that of Glasgow.

All three interpretations presuppose that mortality was related to patterns of urban poverty brought about by the migration and factors antecedent and subsequent to it. This does not preclude the possibility that other health factors were also involved. Changes in real income do not always relate well to changes in health, and medical, hygienic and epidemiological factors need consideration as well (Schofield *et al.* 1991). But urban poverty was associated with enough medically significant factors in the last century – poor nutrition, overcrowding, poor clothing and heating, restricted access to clean water, poor hygiene, frequent adverse life events, and so on – to make it an intelligible basis for mortality predictions.

All these interpretations also predict that high mortality was especially characteristic of cities and regions like Glasgow and Clydeside to which large numbers of peasant immigrants came. This hypothesis is the most important one to emerge here, though it will have to be tested elsewhere. Meanwhile, by distinguishing between these three interpretations of peasant emigration to the cities, it is also possible to formulate differing hypotheses about the duration of those cities' health disadvantage. These two issues – how patterns of urban poverty arose, and what duration of ill health they implied – are the concern of this section.

What was particular, as regards patterns of poverty, about emigration from peasant areas rather than from areas of agricultural capitalism? For purposes of comparison, we may start with a standard neoclassical account of the relation between agriculture and industrialization, of a kind which has been proposed for the largely non-peasant rural population of England. According to this view, with allowance for occasional imperfections and delays in the market, the increase in population led to rises in food prices, which in turn enabled landlords to invest in agricultural productivity sufficiently to feed the whole rising population, and at the same time to employ the same agricultural labour force, though not that part of it which constituted the population increase. Concurrently, capital formation, not least among landlords, together with other factors like the growth of markets, enabled investments to be made also in industrial productivity, whence industrial wages rose, attracting the surplus population from the countryside (Chambers and Mingay 1966). Essential to this view is the assumption that there was no forced reduction of the agricultural labour force and no forced deterioration in their conditions, and that there were no significant losses experienced by migrants to industrial towns, including in health, which might offset their rise in wages.

Now it is already apparent that, while the neoclassical account appears to do well enough with many aspects of the English experience, it cannot explain the experience of the classic peasant areas. In Ireland and Wales, and to some extent in the Highlands, as I noted earlier, the agricultural population did not remain constant as productivity improved, but fell drastically after 1841. Similarly the deterioration in conditions marked by famine, already discussed, argues against emigration being the result of the simple attraction of higher industrial wages in an agricultural economy which was able to feed, but not to employ, an increasing population.

As a result, historians who in other respects are broadly sympathetic with the neoclassical approach, have in Ireland and elsewhere tended to supplement it with elements of a Malthusian account, following Clapham, who declared bluntly that high Irish mortality was inevitable and without the immigration would have been worse: 'If skill had not increased in England,' as he put it, 'the Irish would have died in Ireland' (Clapham 1926:57n). Although Malthus formulated his theory of food resource limits to population growth at the very point when industrialism was in general about to transcend it, it remains possible to apply it in specific circumstances. Because industrial resources such as minerals were limited in Ireland and the Highlands, though not in Wales, the scope for industrialization was more restricted there, and the principal local alternative to agriculture in these areas in the early nineteenth century – the textile industry – had in any case lost its competitive edge due to innovations in Lancashire and Yorkshire at the very period when the market slumped following the high prices of the Napoleonic Wars (Cullen 1972; Cullen and Smout 1978). In these circumstances, population growth was likely to encounter the Malthusian checks. And even if agricultural improvement was occurring without industrial development, the checks were bound to impose themselves if no way was devised of distributing the agricultural product to the population at large through welfare schemes or the like. According to this view, then, the substantial population growth in Ireland and the Highlands in the early nineteenth century, which, in so far as it evoked attempts at preventive restraint, was restrained too late, led inevitably to the last of the classic subsistence famines, impoverishing the peasantry in both areas, and in Ireland, owing to the primitive state of the Poor Law, bringing catastrophic mortality.

The health implications of this interpretation are substantial. From this perspective, we would expect a crisis of poverty and mortality both among those who remained in these areas and among migrants who would have been compelled to find what chances of survival they could in British industrial developments. Virtually any industrial wage would at first have been sufficient for them, and this would have brought down industrial wages generally for a time, but as industrial production expanded to accommodate the larger labour force, so wages would have begun rising again for all workers, whether they were originally from the peasant areas or not. Likewise, the arrival of numbers of destitute peasants would have caused a housing crisis which could not be met until wages rose again, and it would have been in danger of causing a temporary collapse in any system of welfare.

How long a health crisis of this sort would have lasted is hard to say, but seventeenth and eighteenth century examples suggest that starvation and epidemics swept rapidly through a population in this condition, and after a sudden and severe crisis there was an equally rapid return to average or even low mortality (Wrigley and Schofield 1981; Flinn 1977). Thus once over, there is no particular reason on Malthusian or neoclassical grounds for supposing that it would have left any legacy behind it.

Now it is certainly true that the Irish and Highland potato famine of 1845–9 – not the only famine of the period, but incomparably the worst – is a factor to be considered in the health of Glasgow. The sharp peak of Glasgow mortality around 1851, already shown in Figure 4, is doubtless related at least to the famine in Ireland, where relief was poorly coordinated. What this cannot explain, though, is the intense pressure on housing, the stasis in real incomes, and the steep rise in mortality over the whole period between 1821 and 1851. For this, a long-run, grumbling Malthusian problem has to be invoked, like that suggested by Flinn for the Highlands, from the end of the Napoleonic Wars to the great famine (Flinn 1978). On this interpretation, there was just sufficient preventive reaction, initially by emigration to the armed forces and elsewhere, and latterly by well-organized famine relief as well (though not in Ireland), to stop the Malthusian problem from erupting into a crisis, though at the cost of a general level of impoverishment over several decades. Even if we accept, though, that an underlying Malthusian problem caused a certain level of poverty and emigration in Ireland and the Highlands over a long period, the crucial question here is whether this was sufficient to lead to worse health in these areas. A comparison between mortality in industrial cities and in peasant areas is essential.

However, although the Malthusian account has long been a favourite way of accounting for the Irish experience in particular, not all historians accept it, and Joel Mokyr is one who has recently assembled some impressive demographic and economic evidence against it (Mokyr 1983). One alternative lies in those views which presuppose some form of continuing economic maldistribution or exploitation, represented by nineteenth-century critics like Cobbett, Marx and Morris, and by twentieth-century critics like the Hammonds, Hobsbawm and E.P. Thompson. This is a long and diverse tradition, later extended by a literature on contemporary labour migration (Castles and Kosack 1985), in which the Irish case has been used as a paradigm of the means by which nineteenth-century capitalism divided and exploited the working class (Miles 1982:ch. 12; cp. Thompson 1963:ch. 12). Here I summarize a few selected elements from various of these sources which are especially relevant to the health of peasant emigrants in the last century.

The first common contention in these alternative accounts is that exploitation occurred wherever the potential for improved farming methods caused labour to be turned off the land. The argument is obviously strongest wherever there were at the same time blocks to the development of other industries in the area. In this case, landlords who could sustain output with reduced labour stood to gain in a zero sum game where labour had little in the way of economic alternatives. The possibility of such a situation has to be considered wherever violent resistance successfully opposed evictions, or, in so far as this failed, where there was impoverishment, adoption of marginal subsistence methods, or, for those who could afford it, emigration. In this situation, emigrants might not be as poor as their fellows, but being without alternatives at home they would accept a much lower industrial wage than peasants operating in a perfect neoclassical market. The same conditions would then obtain, though less severe and over a longer period, as in a Malthusian crisis, with a depression of industrial wages and of the industrial cities' housing market and welfare system; and at the same time opportunities would occur for continuing maldistribution of economic benefits in the industrial areas. A situation in which labour is made cheap by exploitation in the agricultural sector, or even, if the Malthusian case is correct, by famine in the agricultural sector, weakens its bargaining power in the industrial sector, reducing checks to monopsonistic practices by industrial employers, and making it possible for them to compete by driving down wages instead of investing locally and increasing productivity. The welfare system must also, of course, be made more deterrent if this process is to be successful. And the result, from a neoclassical point of view, is very imperfect market behaviour, for the local consumer market is also impoverished, the housing industry is severely limited, and service industry finds it difficult to expand. How long and to what extent this vicious circle would be maintained is again hard to say, but it seems clear that it could have lasted much longer than the effects of a Malthusian crisis, in fact at least until the rise of organized labour and the welfare state; and its consequences in slow-moving markets like that for housing, could be especially protracted.

The health effects of all this are easy to imagine. The pattern of poverty thus predicted would be consistent, through the mechanisms mentioned earlier, with relatively severe and prolonged health problems, possibly in the peasant areas themselves, but more probably, because of the serial accumulation of adverse circumstances, in the cities to which peasants emigrated. These cities could, as a result, be expected to have worse health than other cities, and to sustain this pattern, again, at least until the rise of organized labour and the welfare state.

In this context, there is certainly evidence for attempts by both Irish and Highland landlords, more intensely opposed in Ireland, to consolidate land and evict tenants long before the famine (Mokyr 1983:ch. 5; Hoppen 1989:44–50; Richards 1982). There is evidence, as I have noted, that the cottage textile industry in Ireland was simultaneously collapsing in many areas and that other Irish industry was slow in developing (Cullen 1972:ch. 5). There is also evidence for monopsonistic practices among British employers in the mining and construction industries, who extensively used Irish labour, and who on a number of occasions were found to be binding their workforce by manipulation of tied housing and by payment in tokens for company shops instead of money. Similarly, there is evidence for the use of Irish labour to break strikes and hold down wages (Royal Commission 1835; Gallagher 1987; Redford 1976: ch. 8; Clapham 1926:548f). These and other indications make this interpretation look quite fertile, and it is consistent with the sustained period of high mortality in Glasgow from 1831 to 1881, after which public health measures on the one hand, and organized labour on the other, became more effective. But further evidence is needed of sustained high mortality in other industrial cities and regions which could exploit peasant immigrants for this account to be better supported.

Finally, there is a third perspective which is neglected in the primarily economic accounts so far outlined. The particularities of peasant culture need consideration (Shanin 1990:ch. 8). So too does the pre-industrial history of the British state, where Michael Hechter's (1975) work is still of relevance – not so much in his account of contemporary nationalism (Sacouman 1985; Williams 1981), nor in his delineation of contemporary Scotland and Wales as internal colonies of the English crown (Kendrick *et al.* 1985; Hechter 1982; Lovering 1978; Cohn 1982), but in his suggestion that political, cultural and religious factors were deeply involved in forming the national division of labour in the past and well into the present century. Similar issues have also been explored with tantalizing brevity in the debate about Scottish economic development between Smout (1980) and Wallerstein (1980). Here I confine myself to such elements of these arguments as seem relevant to the health of peasant immigrants.

The alliance of establishment Protestantism with British aspirations to national sovereignty over Ireland and Scotland had drastically reconstructed the pattern of ownership in both countries from well before the industrial period – from Cromwellian times in Ireland, and after the watershed of 1688 in both countries. The long shadow of anti-Jacobite and anti-Catholic fear and hostility which governed the British Crown's view of Ireland and the Highlands for the century after 1688 meant the concentration of land ownership among Irish Protestants and a policy of breaking up the Highland clans and absorbing their leaders into the English landowning class. Similarly, Welsh landowners had been Anglicized at an early date. Thus a cultural divide opened up between landowners and the peasantry, and between the peasants and the people of those areas where agricultural and industrial capitalism were dominant, which had the potential to exacerbate at every turn any imperfections in the extent to which the neoclassical model of industrial development was realized.

A number of consequences could have followed from this cultural segregation in the migration to the industrial cities. In the first place, the willingness of the metropolitan centre to channel relief to the victims of agricultural change would depend on the extent to which they were seen as members of the same social body. In this respect, the refusal of the government in London to provide sufficient assistance in Ireland after 1847 is significant (Mokyr 1983). Secondly, peasant culture may well have increased resistance to emigration, the landlords' preferred solution. Freedom to hold and work land is itself often a value among the peasantry, with its own symbolic dimensions, and as a preference for a form of labour, it has to be added as a counteracting factor to any model of mere consumer and income preferences. Consumption is not necessarily maximized if there is a counteracting preference about modes of labour. Similarly, a preference for children over consumer goods is also often characteristic of the peasantry, both because children are a future stock of labour and insure against old age, and also for their own sake. The case is argued for Ireland by Mokyr (1983:60–2). If preferences of this kind were held in the nineteenth-century peasant areas of the British Isles, then a much larger wage difference, or a more formidable duress, would have been needed to attract them to industrial cities than in the case of labourers in the areas of agricultural capitalism. And they would be all the poorer when they came, with health consequences which have already been rehearsed.

Furthermore, once arrived, their cultural segregation would have operated against them in numerous ways. Their values and preferences would tend to be misunderstood and denigrated, they would tend to adopt a defensive subculture, and they would be the more easily labelled as outsiders in any situation of economic competition. Add to that connotations of religious dissidence and political disloyalty (Gallagher 1987:14–15, 250–4; Bruce 1985:24–31; Handley 1947:chap. 4–5), and a self-reinforcing social process would arise in which there was a permanent pecking order of access to economic goods, one which, as the tide of prosperity came in, could fall into abeyance, but as the tide of prosperity ebbed again, could be reactivated as goods and opportunities became scarce (Banton 1983).

These cultural processes are as likely as any to persist indefinitely, and in so far as cultural segregation has continued, we would expect both poverty and ill health also to persist within the ethnic or religious minority descended from peasant immigrants. There are, of course, forces which have acted against their persistence – organized labour, to the extent that it created a common front; the free market, to the extent that it rewarded ability irrespective of social origin; the process of intermarriage, to the extent that the bonds of locality or religion permitted it. But how far these forces have eliminated cultural segregation is a matter for empirical inquiry. The crucial test here is first, whether industrial cities and regions which drew in large quantities of peasant immigrants have retained persistently high mortality, and second, whether this is attributable in any degree to exceptionally high mortality among the embattled subcultures concerned.

Health effects of varying duration, then, may help to discriminate which of these three accounts of peasant immigration most needs investigating. Similarly, the broader linkage suggested by all of them between peasant areas, migration and urban mortality can be tested by an analysis across cities and regions. These health hypotheses cannot be put to the evidence here, and this process will be the subject of a further paper. But I hope at least to have shown that what happened to health is a crucial question in the way we evaluate the industrial revolution; and that the evaluation must also now include a theoretical account of why the rise of industrial cities is linked with what happened to the peasant areas of the British Isles. It is with some reflection on these points that I conclude.

Conclusion

The introduction to this chapter argued that judgements about the industrial revolution vary according to three broad schools of thought, of which the most optimistic is the neoclassical perspective. The essence of this view is that production rose faster than population, both in agriculture and industry, and that market forces were sufficiently well developed to distribute the benefits to the mass of the increasing population in rising real wages and reduced mortality, without the need for forced reductions in the agricultural labour force.

Now the national data which have been presented for the nineteenth century suggest that enough people got richer and healthier to raise the average level; and that fact alone has done much to sustain the popularity of the neoclassical view. But this depends on the nation being interpreted as England and Wales, or rather, since Wales does not bulk large in such company, as England. In Scotland, the experience of Clydeside is in marked contrast, and Clydeside was affected by processes occurring in the Highlands and Ireland. Even neoclassically-minded historians of Ireland and the Highlands have not been able to avoid introducing Malthusian factors into their account. And once Ireland and the Highlands are included, other neighbouring areas of Britain which might otherwise be overlooked as atypical and peripheral, such as Wales, the Lakes and Dales, and north-east Scotland, are seen to have a larger significance.

Clearly, then, assessments of the industrial revolution ought to look at the British Isles as a whole; but this does not mean that we should arrive at still more dubious averages over a still wider area. Rather, it is the difference between two broad regions within the former British Isles which emerges most strikingly. In one region – the smaller in area and population, but as it happens the best documented in economic terms – agricultural capitalism was already well developed by 1850, and it may well be that landless wage workers subjected to an authoritarian hierarchy were eager to obtain the better wages and greater freedom of life in commercial and administrative centres. In the other larger region – poorly documented in economic terms, but more equally documented in terms of health – various forms of peasant economy formed the aspirations of the mass of the people, but population growth together with an export sector responsive to commercial opportunities was forcing more and more people to the margins of the land or directly into emigration, and the resulting outflow of broken peasants from many areas was a major factor in the rise of industrial cities.

If this is true, any judgement on the industrial revolution as such must be concerned principally with the industrial cities and their recruiting grounds. The wider growth of the market is certainly not irrelevant, for that helped to create the conditions for industrial growth. Similarly the market enabled commercial areas to reap the benefits of cheap manufactures without necessarily paying the costs. But by the same token, for any attempt to examine the costs of industrial growth, the industrial areas and their recruiting grounds are the point of departure.

In these industrial regions and their hinterland, health may be one of the best measures of what happened, though it must obviously be used circumspectly. Alternative explanations such as the influence of medical and hygienic developments need to be compared with the evidence for economic influences before we accept too readily that health reflected economic change (Williams 1990). But the initial explorations reported here suggest that in Britain's industrial regions and their peasant recruiting grounds, there may well have been a catastrophic immiseration, one to which population increase, local constraints on industrial development, patterns of maldistribution and exploitation, and patterns of cultural segregation may all have contributed. The extent and spread of this catastrophe needs now to be carefully assessed.

Appendix

The Irish Census of 1851 shows a ratio of 49 per cent between male farmers and men who were farmer's labourers, servants and ploughmen.

We meet here a problem of defining 'farmers' that bedevilled the census both in Ireland and, to a lesser extent, in the Scottish Highlands – both places incomprehensible to the liberal economists who presided over industrializing England. Nassau Senior said of Ireland that there were people there '*called* landlords, farmers and labourers, but they resemble their English types in little but name' (Fitzpatrick 1980:67). The Irish 'agricultural labourer' was a figment of the landlords' and the baffled census takers' assumptions, for those so named often refused this title and called themselves 'landholders' instead, and correspondingly often held land, or were younger members of a family which held land (*ibid.* 67, 68–9, 72, 76–7) – both clear marks, from the present point of view, of peasants, in this case poor peasants, who cannot maintain themselves entirely off their land, or at any rate not while also paying rent, and must therefore send some family members to work for their rent or additional subsistence for at least part of the year.

How self-subsistent were Ireland's 'agricultural labourers' or poor peasants in the early nineteenth century? The question is obviously material to any comparison with the rest of Britain. Fitzpatrick, whose thorough study of the nineteenth-century Irish census materials is fundamental on the history of the labourer, unfortunately answers this question by assumption. Observing that the census distinction between 'farmer' and 'labourer' was at least remarkably consistent over decades, he suggests that the basis for the judgement was that 'farmers' maintained themselves mainly from the produce of their own farms while 'farm workers' earned most of their livelihood by working for 'farmers' (*ibid.* 70). It is, however, just as possible, and it would be a simpler coding decision, that 'farm workers' were those who earned *any* part of their livelihood, or perhaps paid any part of their rent, by working for 'farmers'. It is worth noting that the number of male 'farmers' in 1851 was slightly smaller than the number of farms over ten acres in the Devon Commission's report of 1845, and a ten acre minimum for 'farmers' is also consistent with the 1851 data on number and size of holdings, though sizes are not broken down so finely (Mokyr 1983:19; Census of Ireland 1851, Agriculture:v, cp. General Report: Farmers). If a dozen acres was enough for subsistence in corn country (Chambers and Mingay 1966:21), among German peasants (Clapham 1926:110), or as the gift of a grateful government to First World War heroes in the Outer Hebrides (Macdonald 1983:ch. 1), then more than ten would surely be enough in nineteenth-century potato country, and Irish 'farmers' in this case were fully self-subsistent, and possibly able to pay the rent as well. Correspondingly, 'labourers' must have been those who engaged in any labour for subsistence, and possibly in any labour in lieu of rent.

The Irish agricultural labourer, then, will often, by the frugal standards of the time, have been a relatively self-sufficient figure compared with the landless English labourer. Therefore, instead of counting 'farmers', I have estimated *all* occupiers of over an acre of land in 1851 (Fitzpatrick 1980:72 and n.20), and subtracted the excess of occupiers over 'farmers' from the 'labourer' figures, thus obtaining the ratio of landholders to labour of 79 per cent in Table 1.

In the Scottish Highlands, meanwhile, a similar problem of classification was encountered with those who called themselves 'crofters', but whose acreage was unstated or, in the census takers' opinion, 'very inconsiderable' (Census of Scotland 1851, vol. 2.2:909n.). In 1851 these were allocated to 'agricultural labourers (outdoor)', but by 1861 many of them were evidently reinstated as 'farmers', and this remained so thereafter. In Orkney and Shetland, for example, the population of male farmers and labourers together barely changed between 1851 and 1861, yet male farmers and graziers rose from 1,013 to 3,576, and male farm servants and labourers shrank from 4,400 to 2,147. No doubt some of these changes were due to the acreages of 'farmers' being better documented by 1861, but a substantial part must have been due to a reclassification of 'crofters'. In 1901, when crofters were first classified separately, the number of male farmers and crofters together in Orkney and Shetland was still much the same as that of male farmers in 1861, and crofters formed 38 per cent of the total (Census of Scotland 1861, vol. 2:141; Census of Scotland 1901, vol. 3:24, 31). Similar large shifts in the farmer figures between 1851 and 1861 occurred in Inverness, Argyll and Sutherland, all later identified as crofting counties.

A rough correction can be made for this problem in the 1851 farmer figures by taking the difference between them and the 1861 farmer figures in the counties concerned, and by subtracting this residue of false 'labourers' from the 1851 labourer figures. When this is done, the number of farmers (including crofters) in the Highlands is 72 per cent of the number of labourers – a result very similar to that for Ireland.

Acknowledgements

I am grateful to Andrew Findlay, Sally Macintyre and Kenneth Mullen for helpful comments on this chapter, and to Jacqui Irwin for typing the original manuscript.

Note

1. In 1851 Glasgow had 13.2 per cent under 5 and 2.4 per cent aged 65 and over, while England and Wales had 13.4 per cent and 4.6 per cent respectively. In decades before and after, the former comparison varied, the latter remained stable. However changes in the size of the under 5 age group do not affect the

issue, since in Glasgow the proportion under 5 declined during 1821–51 when the crude death rate was rising, and rose from 1851–61 when the crude death rate fell.

References

Banton, M. (1983), *Racial and ethnic competition*, Cambridge: Cambridge University Press.

Bruce, S. (1985), *No Pope of Rome: Anti-Catholicism in Modern Scotland*, Edinburgh: Mainstream.

Cage, R.A. (1983), 'The standard of living debate: Glasgow 1800–1850', *Journal of Economic History*, **43**:175–182.

Cage, R.A. (1987), 'The standard of living debate', in Cage, R.A. (ed.), *The working class in Glasgow 1750–1914*, London: Croom Helm.

Carter, I.R. (1979), *Farm Life in North-East Scotland 1840–1914: The Poor Man's Country*, Edinburgh: Donald.

Castles, S. and Kosack, G. (1985), *Immigrant Workers and Class Structure in Western Europe*, 2nd edn, Oxford: Oxford University Press.

Census of Great Britain (1821), London: HMSO.

Census of Great Britain (1851), Edinburgh: HMSO.

Census of Ireland (1851), Dublin: HMSO.

Census of Scotland (1861), Edinburgh: HMSO.

Census of Scotland (1901), Edinburgh: HMSO.

Census of England and Wales (1901), London: HMSO.

Census of England and Wales (1911), London: HMSO.

Census of Scotland (1911), Edinburgh: HMSO.

Chambers, J.D. and Mingay, G.E. (1966), *The Agricultural Revolution 1750–1880*, London: Batsford.

Clapham, J.H. (1926), *The Economic History of Modern Britain, Volume 1: The Early Railway Age*, Cambridge: Cambridge University Press.

Cohn, S. (1982), 'Michael Hechter's theory of regional underdevelopment: a test case using Victorian railways', *American Sociological Review*, **47**:477–488.

Cullen, L.M. (1972), *An Economic History of Ireland Since 1660*, London: Batsford.

Cullen, L.M. and Smout, T.C. (1978), 'Economic growth in Scotland and Ireland', in Cullen, L.M. and Smout, T.C. (eds), *Comparative Aspects of Scottish and Irish Economic and Social History 1600–1900*, Edinburgh: Donald.

de Vries, J. (1984), *European Urbanisation 1500–1800*, London: Methuen.

Fitzpatrick, D. (1980), 'The disappearance of the Irish agricultural labourer', *Irish Economic and Social History*, **7**:66–92.

Flinn, M. (ed.) (1977), *Scottish Population History from the 17th Century to the 1930s*, Cambridge: Cambridge University Press.

Flinn, M.W. (1978), 'Emigration and potatoes in the Scottish north-west 1770–1870', in Cullen, L.M. and Smout, T.C. (eds), *Comparative Aspects of Scottish and Irish Economic and Social History 1600–1900*, Edinburgh: Donald.

Floud, R., Wachter, K. and Gregory, A. (1990), *Height, Health and History*, Cambridge: Cambridge University Press.

Friedlander, D. and Roshier, R.J. (1966a), 'A study of internal migration in England and Wales: part 1', *Population Studies*, **19**:239–279.
Friedlander, D. and Roshier, R.J. (1966b), 'A study of internal migration in England and Wales: part 2', *Population Studies*, **19**:239–279.
Gallagher, T. (1987), *Glasgow – The Uneasy Peace: Religious Tension in Modern Scotland 1819–1914*, Manchester: Manchester University Press.
Gilboy, E.W. (1975), 'The cost of living and real wages in eighteenth-century England', in Taylor, A.J. (ed.), *The Standard of Living in Britain in the Industrial Revolution*, London: Methuen.
Handley, J.E. (1947), *The Irish in Modern Scotland*, Cork: Cork University Press.
Hechter, M. (1975), *Internal Colonialism: The Celtic Fringe in British National Development 1536–1966*, London: Routledge.
Hechter, M. (1982), '"Internal colonialism" revisited', *Cencrastus* (autumn).
Hoppen, K.T. (1989), *Ireland Since 1800: Conflict and Conformity*, London: Longman.
Howell, D.W. (1977), *Land and People in Nineteenth-Century Wales*, London: Routledge.
Kendrick, S., Bechhofer, F. and McCrone, D. (1985), 'Is Scotland different? Industrial and occupational change in Scotland and Britain', in Newby, H., Bujra, J., Littlewood, P., Rees, G. and Rees, T.L. (eds), *Restructuring Capital: Recession and Reorganisation in Industrial Society*, London: Macmillan.
Lovering, J. (1978), 'The theory of the "internal colony" and the political economy of Wales', *Review of Radical Political Economics*, **10**:55–67.
Miles, R. (1982), *Racism and Migrant Labour*, London: Routledge.
Mokyr, J. (1983), *Why Ireland Starved: A Quantitative and Analytical History of the Irish Economy 1800–1850*, London: Allen and Unwin.
Macdonald, F.J. (1983), *Crowdie and Cream: Memoirs of a Hebridean Childhood*, London: Futura.
Macfarlane, A. (1978), *The Origins of English Individualism*, Oxford: Blackwell.
O'Grada, C. (1975), 'A note on nineteenth-century Irish emigration statistics', *Population Studies*, **29**:143–9.
O'Grada, C. (1978), 'Some aspects of nineteenth-century Irish emigration', in Cullen, L.M. and Smout, T.C. (eds), *Comparative Aspects of Scottish and Irish Economic and Social History 1600–1900*, Edinburgh: Donald.
Redford, A. (1976), *Labour Migration in England 1800–1850*, 3rd edn, Manchester: Manchester University Press.
Richards, E. (1982), *A History of the Highland Clearances*, London: Croom Helm.
Royal Commission (1835), *Royal Commission on the Conditions of the Poorer Classes in Ireland*, Appendix G: The state of the Irish poor in Great Britain, Parliamentary Papers Vol. xxxiv, (40).
Sacouman, R.J. (1985), 'Broken-up Canada and breaking-up Britain: some comparative lessons in uneven development, regionalism and nationalism during the current crisis', in Rees, G., Bujra, J., Littlewood, P., Newby, H. and Rees, T.L. (eds), *Political Action and Social Identity*, London: Macmillan.
Schofield, R., Reher, D. and Bideau, A. (eds) (1991), *The Decline of Mortality in Europe*, Oxford: Oxford University Press.
Shanin, T. (1990), *Defining Peasants*, Oxford: Blackwell.

Sinclair, Sir John (1795), *The Statistical Account of Scotland, Volume 7*, edited by Withrington, D.J. and Grant, I.R., Wakefield: EP Publishing Co., (1973).
Slaven, A. (1975), *The Development of the West of Scotland 1750–1960*, London: Routledge.
Smout, T.C. (1980), 'Scotland and England: is dependency a symptom or a cause of underdevelopment?', *Review*, **3**:601–630.
Taylor, A.J. (ed.) (1975), *The Standard of Living in Britain in the Industrial Revolution*, London: Methuen.
Thompson, E.P. (1963), *The Making of the English Working Class*, London: Gollancz.
Vaughan, W.E. and Fitzpatrick, A.J. (1978), *Irish Historical Statistics: Population 1821–1971*, Dublin: Royal Irish Academy.
Wallerstein, I. (1980), 'One man's meat: the Scottish Great Leap Forward', *Review*, **3**:631–640.
Williams, G. (1981), 'Economic development, social structure, and contemporary nationalism in Wales', *Review*, **5**:275–310.
Williams, R. (1990), 'Glasgow: the evolving health of a city', paper presented to the Society for Social Medicine Conference, Glasgow.
Wrigley, E.A. and Schofield, R.S. (1981), *The Population History of England 1541–1871: A Reconstruction*, Cambridge: Cambridge University Press.

11 'Keeping up with the Joneses?' Private health insurance as a consumption good?

Michael Calnan, Sarah Cant and Jonathan Gabe

Several writers (Dunleavy and Husbands, 1985; Saunders 1978, 1984, 1986, 1990) have argued that social divisions may be more usefully explored by concentrating on divisions associated with the sphere of consumption rather than production. However, there is some disagreement about the relative importance of consumption divisions compared with class divisions. For example, Saunders (1984, 1986) emphasizes that the analysis of social divisions should centre on the dimensions of personal ownership (autonomy and control) which is independent of class divisions. Dunleavy and Husbands (1985), in contrast, suggest an interrelationship between class and consumption, noting that in some situations sectoral divisions cut across class lines, whereas in others they are derived from class divisions. However, both sets of writers agree that divisions in the consumption sector between those people reliant on the state for housing, transport and health and welfare services and those who satisfy their requirements through the private market do shape political attitudes and cultural perceptions.

Much of the discussion around this issue has either been theoretical in nature or based on findings regarding private consumption in the area of housing (Hamnett 1989). In the health field the main contribution has come from Busfield (1990) who has explored the implications of changes in the consumption of health care for social divisions through a secondary analysis of the General Household Survey.

In this chapter the aim is to explore the debate about health care consumption further, on the basis of findings from a study which has recently been undertaken regarding the decision to subscribe to private health insurance and the decision to use it. Three questions are examined which have emerged from the new sociology of consumption. The first of these is whether the decision to opt for a 'privatized form of health provision' (private health insurance) signifies new social divisions which are independent of, or related to class. Closely related to this is whether consumption location shapes political ideologies. The second question focuses on the issue of the 'culture of consumption' and whether the introduction of the market economy into health care not only confers on the 'customer' purchasing power but also autonomy and freedom of choice. For example, is there any evidence of consumers of private health care 'shopping around' for health care? Finally, the third question concerns the cultural significance of private health insurance and whether it is similar to other forms of consumption good? Clearly, certain types of consumer good have a status over and above their material value and this analysis focuses on how private health insurance is perceived in relation to other types of good. Each of these questions is examined in turn before the implications are drawn out for the sociology of consumption debate.

The data

Before these questions can be discussed, it is necessary to describe how the data from the private health insurance study were collected. The methods employed have been discussed in detail elsewhere (Calnan *et al.* 1993) and therefore will only be described briefly here. The data on private insurance subscribers were collected through a two stage method of sampling. The first stage consisted of a postal survey of middle aged men (35 to 55) registered with four general practices in relatively affluent areas of Kent. Of the 3,060 men sampled, 1688 (55 per cent) sent back a completed questionnaire. The study focused primarily on middle aged men, because at the time the study was carried out, they were the largest group of subscribers. However, it is recognized that women also tend to be covered by their partner's subscription although the major focus here was on decisions to subscribe (Nicholl *et al.* 1981).

The questionnaire asked about whether the person was currently subscribing to private health insurance, their use of private health insurance, their socio-political beliefs about the health service; their satisfaction with and patterns of use of the health services, health status and socio-demographic characteristics.

The second stage of the study involved in-depth, semi-structured interviews with small samples of men matched for socio-demographic characteristics who had taken part in the postal survey. They were divided into three groups of equal size (N = 20) according to whether they had

i) personally chosen to take out private health insurance (I);
ii) been co-opted into employer run schemes (Co);
iii) had not subscribed to a scheme (Non).

The sample itself, not surprisingly given the sampling frame, was skewed towards the middle class with 42 per cent coming from the Registrar General's Social Classes 1 and 2 and 61 per cent of subscribers to private health insurance coming from this middle class group. Each of the sixty interviews completed lasted one and a half hours on average and were tape-recorded. The bulk of the data used in the analysis presented here is derived from these qualitative interviews.

A new social cleavage?

Do people who subscribe to private health insurance hold a distinct set of political beliefs and ideologies? In order to throw light on this question, our interviewees were asked about their views on the following issues: private education; private pensions; the selling of council houses; the growth of private homes for the elderly and disabled; privatization of industries, including utilities such as gas and water; and the contracting out of transport cleaning and refuse collection services by local councils. If the sample of subscribers and non-subscribers hold similar views about each of these issues, it would provide grounds for questioning the proposition that private health insurance can be used to explain social divisions, at least in terms of political beliefs and ideologies.

The first part of the analysis focused on identifying the range (if any) of ideologies used by the sample respondents. The second part focused on the variation (if any) by type of subscriber. Three distinct ideologies emerged from the analysis. These stressed: individual responsibility for health and welfare, state responsibility for provision of services, and joint responsibility between state and individual. Each of the three ideologies in turn will be considered.

Individual responsibility and choice

The importance of individual responsibility, choice, and personal control, a value placed on both competition and home ownership and the constraining influence of the state were key elements in this set of ideological beliefs. These aspects are well illustrated below, in the respondents' accounts, beginning with individual initiative, choice and responsibility:

> This government has given the individual initiative. It has been made clear to us that if we want to get on in this life we've got to do the job.(I)

> I'm always a believer that the consumer should be powerful, you know the consumer should be the one to determine what is provided. Health is an unusual commodity isn't it? I should like to think the consumer would be able to

> determine but at the end of the day I don't think they can. How do you judge? You can only do it after the event, but you can choose private. I think I should be permitted within the realms of legality to spend money on what I wish.(Co)

Privatization and competition are illustrated by the following quotes:

> Privatisation means good healthy competition.(I)

> The private sector is efficient, accountable and apolitical.(Co)

The benefits of the privatization of welfare services are illustrated by the following:

> Private education is much better than state education, it offers choice.(I)

> Don't know why we had council houses in the first place, private everything apart from the National Health!(I)

> Private pensions are a great idea, state does not provide enough.(Non)

> Owning your home allows you to be master of your own destiny.(Co)

State responsibility

This ideology identifies the state as entirely responsible for provision of services and determining individual needs. The state is perceived as the most appropriate provider, as health and welfare services are best not left to the market and the state can ensure that the population as a whole receive services and can minimize inequalities. Once again, these different aspects are clearly illustrated in the respondents' accounts beginning with the state portrayed as paternalistic provider:

> The state is responsible for health. I think it is a total shame that all these things that were and are run by the government are being privatised like water, electricity and by the sound of it health. I don't think it is a good idea at all. The idea of a caring state is good. Private companies' idea – to make profits.(Non)

> Government has got to organise health and education because it has to look after the ones who can't take care of themselves. Private poaches off the rest. Selling of council houses is absolutely criminal! You can give people assistance to buy houses but that is politically motivated.(Co)

The next series of quotes illustrate the role of the state in the reduction of inequalities:

> The private sector weakens the public. Privatising education is bad for the community, it splits it up, it stratifies it, it divides it.(Co)

> All the changes just divide rich and poor.(Non)

and the role of the state as the provider of basic needs:

> Health, education and water should be more public than anything else.(I)

> Government should have control of all basics.(Co)

The public/private mix

The third ideological type which emerged through the analysis sees the responsibility for health and welfare as lying with both the state and the individual. It does not designate either the state or the individual as being more important but sees some services as being more applicable for the state to provide than others. This approach is characterized by: (i) a need for joint responsibility as the following respondents' accounts illustrate:

> The individual is primarily responsible, the government is responsible to ensure a system exists. (I)

> It's the state's responsibility to produce the means and it's up to the individual to look after themselves. In a democratic society you have to have both public and private, but the state should be leading the way.(Co)

> We are all responsible, but the state should be responsible too. (Non)

and (ii) a mixed economy in terms of provision:

> Competition if it's not an essential service.(Co)

> Selling council houses? Ok, so long as you build more for those unable to buy.(I)

Classifying the data in this way provides the basis for making the following observations. First, no respondent fitted exactly into any ideology. Instead, they combined strands from at least two of the ideologies during the interview (or while discussing a particular question). Not only was such juggling exhibited in many pro-privatization comments about health, it was also apparent in talk about selling council houses. Again, respondents drew on two or three ideologies simultaneously or used one or the other in responding to different questions. Secondly, holding strands from all three types of ideology did not necessarily mean everyone falls into type three.

The third type of ideology is where the respondent sees the state and private sectors working together simultaneously in specific areas.

Were any of these three types of political ideology more prevalent among one or other of the groups of private health insurance subscribers? Overall, there was not any clear evidence of differences between the groups although subscribers more often referred to individual responsibility than non-subscribers. However, it was in relation to specific issues that differences were more in evidence. While there was general antagonism towards private health care amongst almost the whole sample, irrespective of subscription to private health insurance, differences did emerge in relation to private education. Individual subscribers favoured private education, whereas non-subscribers were fervently anti-private education because it was 'snobbish' and 'divisive'.

In summary, the analysis so far suggests that private health insurance is a weak indicator of new social divisions in that there is little evidence that subscription to private health insurance was associated with a distinct set of political beliefs and ideologies. Certainly, in relation to health care, there appeared to be a consensus amongst the sample as a whole that it was a basic service which the state should provide, although there was less of a consensus about other areas of welfare.

Private health insurance and establishing the patient as 'customer'

The second question examines whether having access to private health care through private health insurance gives consumers choice and autonomy in their pattern of health care use. The data collected in this study enabled this question to be examined in a number of different ways. First, there is the issue of perceived choice, which was addressed by asking the respondents directly about the degree of choice available. The questions asked were, did users choose the specialist and hospital, and of non-users whether they thought such choice was available? Responses to these questions about choice of consultant and hospital largely suggest the choice had been made by the GP.

> I didn't choose hospital or doctor, the GP made the choice.
>
> Doctors are talking about something that most people have little knowledge about anyway.
>
> From experience I shouldn't have any choice. If I want private treatment I'm in the private establishment.

Only five out of 28 users argued they had choice of consultant and hospital. As one of them argued:

> You have a choice of hospital and consultant. I chose the one I felt happier with. I think in the earlier days I used to leave it up to the GP but I think now probably with – the business I spend more time on consideration of this and knowing a lot of people here particularly locally in the medical scene. I'm an avid reader of the medical directory actually to see what qualifications people have got …

The last quotation was the only response of this kind and the respondent was different in that his son had a brain tumour and was under constant treatment. Thus this man had lots of contacts and technical knowledge. Furthermore, his other son was a doctor.

In terms of choice of time, more positive responses were given and it was in the context of timing that choice was most clearly articulated:

> Choice is getting something done quicker.

> It's the immediacy of response that is important.

Thus, again speed and timing and jumping the queue are the most important criteria for the respondents. It is interesting to note that the choice of consultant and hospital was rarely mentioned voluntarily. Rather, it was only in response to direct questioning and then in a negative way, suggesting choice in these terms was not an important issue or a reality. Thus, choice was absent from the respondents' discourse, except in relation to timing and speed.

Non-users and non-subscribers were turned to next, to illicit what they thought about choice in the private sector:

> I would expect people to dance if I went private. I demand good service when I am 'shopping' and were I in need of an operation I am 'shopping', there's no difference. In principle I would expect people to jump around and look interested.

It was argued by one non-subscriber that choice was available on the NHS, if you demanded it:

> You can get choice in the NHS if you ask. I think it is a lot easier to choose a time but people are frightened to ask.

Likewise a company subscriber suggested:

> It doesn't make me feel more of a customer. I pay my NI and I am a customer and I am just as entitled to that care ... by being a paying member of the NHS as I am by being private.

Again choice of consultant and hospital was not a noted advantage of the private sector. Non-respondents did not talk in terms of 'choice' in any way except timing. The private sector then confers choice but only in terms of timing.

Secondly, there is the question of the actual pattern of utilization behaviour which shows that, in reality, choice is rather limited. In a previous paper (Cant and Calnan 1992) it was shown that respondents tended to use one sector or the other and there was little evidence of respondents using a mix of both sectors. However, shopping around was evident, at least, in terms of decision-making. Patients did weigh up the advantages and disadvantages of the different options, although it was not manifest in actual behaviour in that many consistently chose in the same way. Resource concerns (such as time and money) were the major criteria on which decisions were made. Also, as was suggested previously, patients are largely referred to private medical care by GPs and in terms of decision-making, the role of the GP is fundamental in influencing patients' pathways to private health care. For many subscribers, then, private medical insurance clearly did not confer autonomy and power. Rather, advice from medical personnel was more influential. This may be due to the special qualities associated with health care, such as the inadequate knowledge base of respondents, or it may be that illness itself can induce passivity. Higgins (1988) also points out that patients' choice of hospital and consultant is limited in that the patient may choose the hospital or the consultant but not both.

The study also highlights other constraints on choice. One of these was the lack of knowledge expressed by the subscribers about the costs of treatment and the extent to which this limited the care covered by the policy. Subscribers, then, do not appear to have the information which would empower them to be an 'enterprising' and 'critical' consumer. In addition, evidence presented previously (Calnan and Cant 1992) suggests that the decision to take out private health insurance was not always an individual choice but a 'perk' or gift bestowed by employers.

Private health insurance as a consumption good

This third section is designed to ascertain whether private health insurance can be designated as a consumption good. It has been argued (Titmuss 1976) that medical care is qualitatively different from other types of goods which are purchased in the market context, because prospective users have no way of knowing how much medical care will be needed in the future. This question was not addressed directly in the study, although the data sheds some light on whether medical care provided by private health insurance has distinctive qualities or whether it is similar to other consumption goods. More specifically, respondents' accounts were examined in terms of the following:

i) Status of private health insurance as a consumer good.
ii) Status of the person who subscribes to private health insurance.
iii) Value attached to private health insurance.
iv) Value attached to private health insurance compared with other consumption goods.

Each of these issues is important in that it gives clues to the social weight and value placed on private health insurance as perceived by the respondents and, thereby, the extent to which it may be defined as a consumption good.

Private health insurance as a status symbol

There was no evidence of a widespread belief amongst the sample that private health insurance was a status symbol. Some suggested that it had once been so, but deemed that this was no longer the case because of it now being more widely available:

> I don't think it's a status symbol, plenty of working class people have it.(I)

For some people it even had negative connotations:

> I wouldn't see it as a status symbol. I'd feel guilty about it.(Non)

The minority who did regard private health insurance as a status symbol tended to be non-subscribers:

> Yes it is. It's a nice thing to drop into conversation, I'd like to meet you but I'm off to my clinic for my annual health check.

Those that did subscribe did not see it as a status symbol for themselves but recognized it could have this potential in the eyes of others:

> Some people have it for status, keeping up with the Joneses.

> It is a status symbol, as well as a lot of other things. Some of my colleagues at work who weren't in private medicine prior to last year when the present

company gave us insurance used to say, it's terrible. The moment it was paid for by the company they rushed at it and I think they regard it as slightly, how shall I put it, one up on the guy next door who can't afford it.

In summary, there was ambivalence about the status of private health insurance. Although subscribers and non-subscribers said that it had a social value, they were negative about those who adhered to this status.

Type of person who is a subscriber

The status of a consumption good appears to be associated not only with the nature of the commodity itself but also with 'the type of person' who purchases it. Was there any evidence of such a stereotyped image (either positive or negative) as being associated with private health insurance? A large number said it was impossible to identify such a typical person nowadays because of the wide social spectrum of people who are subscribers:

I don't associate private health insurance with anyone.
I'm just a normal working guy.(I)

Others, however, felt it was still possible to identify a type of person and distinguished them on grounds such as socio-economic group membership, political values and principles and the importance attached to health.

I associate it with financially stable people, professional rather than industrial. (Co)

Those that take it out are those with a priority for health, not necessarily wealthy. You can make economies if you want to.(I)

Thus, despite the increase in the numbers and 'range' of people holding insurance, it was possible for the respondents to identify certain characteristics of typical holders and non-holders of insurance. Interestingly, these data suggest the need to be cautious about drawing conclusions about private health insurance as a status symbol as they show that a number of the respondents felt 'class' was important and incorporated status type arguments into their responses. Thus, at a public level respondents may state that private health insurance has little importance as a status symbol whereas at the private level, in unstructured discourse, its status connotations may be more apparent.

Private health insurance as a luxury or necessity

What value did those participating in the research place on private health insurance? In this section, responses to a question about whether private health insurance is a luxury or necessity are described. This should give clues as to whether private health insurance is seen as a commodity.

The evidence shows that respondents had different perceptions of the value of private health insurance, according to whether they were subscribers or not. Individual subscribers were the only respondents to describe private health insurance as entirely a necessity:

> I look upon it as a necessity as I'm the breadwinner.

The other two groups were more likely to see private health insurance as a luxury.

> Oh it is a luxury, definitely a luxury. I could happily exist and bring up my family without it.(Co)

However, some were doubtful about the distinction between luxury and necessity.

> It's not a luxury or necessity, it's convenience.(Co)

> It's not a luxury you skimp and save for – it's not a necessity either. You get reasonable treatment in the NHS ... It's almost like a conscious investment.(Co)

Perceptions of the value placed on private health insurance is, according to this evidence, clearly shaped by whether the respondent is personally a subscriber or not. Clearly, for the individual subscriber material interests (such as, being self-employed) shape the meaning attached to it, in that private health insurance is like any other commodity which influences their material circumstances.

The substitutability of private health insurance

In this final section the value put on private health insurance is examined in terms of what the subscribers would give up to continue to subscribe to it. This involves looking at whether other goods would be substituted in favour of private health insurance and what sort of goods these would be.

Not surprisingly, the value placed on private health insurance as a luxury or necessity shaped respondents' perceptions of its substitutability. Those individual subscribers who had described private health insurance as a necessity were prepared to make 'sacrifices' to continue use.

> I would sacrifice most things to keep insurance except school fees. For example, continental holidays … it's a necessity.

> If it (premium) increased dramatically it would go, but I would forego luxuries like a holiday abroad … it's essential.

Individual subscribers who saw private health insurance as a luxury, however, said they might forego spending on certain items although they clearly valued it less.

> I think it's a luxury personally. I would forego spending on one or two meals out, I don't think I would spend less on my holiday because that's important for health reasons.

The majority of company subscribers said they would not forego spending for private health insurance, or substitute it for another good. Indeed, many said they had not wanted it in the first place but that it had been given to them and so they had taken it.

> I would drop it. I wouldn't look for it in a new job, I'd prefer a better pension.

Non-subscribers were asked what they would spend any extra money on and the majority did not identify private health insurance as being desirable.

> If you've got money it's the sort of thing you invest in, but I'd buy other things first.

In summary, the desirability of private health insurance as a 'consumption good' is clearly dependent upon an individual's priorities and the meaning health insurance holds for him (or her). Only for individual subscribers was it seen as a necessity and as something which would not be willingly substituted. For the remainder of the sample, private health insurance was seen as a good which had some attractions but was not seen as being necessary to meet immediate needs.

Discussion

The aim of the empirical analysis described in this paper has been to use private health insurance to throw some light on a number of propositions which have emerged recently amongst proponents of the sociology of consumption. One of the most important propositions adopted by commentators has been that social divisions may be more usefully explored by concentrating on divisions associated with the sphere of consumption rather than production. This approach to the 'new' social divisions has been questioned by, amongst others, Hamnett (1989) who argues that 'class' still has explanatory power at the aggregate level, if not in individual cases. The qualitative research reported here, while not enabling an examination of the 'class' question directly in terms of class-related beliefs, has revealed specific intra-class beliefs and values associated with the 'consumption' of private health insurance.

A number of observations emerged from the analysis, which have implications for the debate about a new social cleavage. The first is that consumption of private health insurance has little power to explain or account for the 'new' social divisions. While there was evidence in respondents' accounts of support for the values associated with 'the new right' ideology (Harris and Seldon 1987), the use of this ideology was not confined to subscribers to private health insurance. In fact, there was evidence that respondents 'juggled' with more than one type of ideology, and the use of ideology seemed to be related to specific issues. Certainly, respondents tended not to operate with a 'new right' or a mixed economy ideology when they discussed the topic of health care. This appears to confirm the view that health and health care have special qualities (Titmuss 1976) that distinguish them from other services and goods. It also explains why subscribers tended to express different ideological views to non-subscribers when discussing other welfare issues.

Second, it is possible to comment on another proposition from the new sociology of consumption which sees privatized forms of service delivery enabling a change in the status of the health service use from passive patient to active, enterprising customer. Saunders and Harris (1990) have argued that only marketization and commodification forms have this quality, and recognized that these forms were underdeveloped. However, little evidence was found in the study reported here, at least as regards private health care, to support any marked increase in the availability of choice, autonomy and freedom. The majority of respondents, whilst feeling they gained an increase in choice in terms of timing as well as more individualized care, did not feel more empowered or more knowledgeable, and there was little evidence of the enterprising customer 'shopping' around. Thus, choice might be expressed in theory but not in the actual health service utilization patterns of the users. However, the evidence presented here was limited to men and further analysis will include women's pattern of utilization, as they tend to be heavier users of private health care.

Finally, the analysis casts light on the status and value attached to private health insurance as a consumption good. The evidence shows that private health insurance, as perceived by respondents, had a social significance over and above its function. Despite denials of status connotations for themselves, respondents tended to describe insurance in social terms. These data suggest that particular beliefs and values are associated with private health care but they also highlight the relationship between private health insurance and class, income and occupation. One implication of this is that the consumption of private health care might be a symbol of socio-economic position rather than a substitute for it.

In conclusion, the evidence from this study adds weight to the claims of those who have argued that private medical care challenges the proposition that divisions of consumption have replaced divisions of production. Busfield (1990) argues that theories of consumption are of little value on the grounds that most people are both private and public consumers of health care. This study provides some support for Busfield's argument, although the level of commuting between similar services in the NHS and private sector was not high. Furthermore, the data suggest that beliefs and ideologies about health care are consistent across subscribers and non-subscribers. They also show that consumption of private health care is associated with images of class and status, suggesting that it may be more useful to see private health insurance as an indicator of social class rather than a substitute for it.

Acknowledgements

This research was funded by a grant from the ESRC. Thanks to Lou Opit for help with setting the study up.

References

Busfield, J. (1990), 'Sectoral divisions and consumption, the case of medical care', *Sociology*, **24**,(1): 77–97.

Calnan, M. and Cant, S.L. (1992), 'Principles and practice: the case of private health insurance', in Burrows, R. and Marsh, C. (eds), *Consumption and Class Divisions and Change*, London: Macmillan, pp. 89–121.

Calnan, M., Cant, S. and Gabe, J. (1993), *Going Private: Why People Pay for their Health Care*, Milton Keynes: Open University Press.

Cant, S.L. and Calnan, M. (1992), 'Using private health insurance', *Sociology of Health and Illness*, **14**,(1): 39–56.

Dunleavy, P. and Husbands, C.T. (1985), *British Democracy at the Crossroads*, London: Allen and Unwin.

Hamnett, C. (1989), 'Consumption and class and contemporary Britain', in Hamnett, C. *et al.* (eds), *The Changing Social Structure*, London: Sage.

Harris, R. and Seldon, A. (1987), *Welfare Without the State. A Quarter Century of Suppressed Public Choice*, Hobart Paperback No. 26, London: Institute of Economic Affairs.

Higgins, J. (1988), *The Business of Medicine*, London: Macmillan.

Nicholl, J., Beeby, N. and Williams, B. (1989), 'Comparison of the activity of short stay independent hospitals in England and Wales 1981 and 1986', *British Medical Journal*, **298**:239–47.

Saunders, P. (1978), 'Domestic property and social class', *International Journal of Urban and Regional Research*, **2**:233–51.
Saunders, P. (1984), 'Beyond housing classes; the sociological significance of private property rights in means of consumption', *International Journal of Urban and Regional Research*, **8**(2): 202–27.
Saunders, P. (1986), *Social Theory and the Urban Question*, London: Hutchinson.
Saunders, P. and Harris, C. (1990), 'Privatization and the consumer', *Sociology*, **24**(1): 57–77.
Titmuss, R. (1976), *Commitment to Welfare*, 2nd edn, London: Allen and Unwin.

12 Health and ignorance: Past and present

David Smith and Malcolm Nicolson

Introduction

In September 1986, Mrs Edwina Currie, the newly appointed Junior Minister at the Department of Health, visited Newcastle. During the course of her visit, she was questioned about the *Interim Report on Inequalities in Health in the Northern Region* (Townsend *et al.* 1986) which had just been published and which pointed to the existence of above average levels of morbidity and mortality in the North of England.[1] Her reply was that 'The problem very often for many people is, I think, just ignorance ...'.[2] She was shortly to expand these remarks with critical observations upon the lifestyle and, especially, the diet of Northerners.[3]

In the last decade or so, the phenomenon of health inequality, its nature, causes and possible cures, has received a great deal of attention from medical sociologists.[4] The intention of the present authors is not to contribute fresh evidence or new methods to this formidable and admirable research effort but to try to put certain aspects of the recent debates about inequalities in health into a broader historical perspective. Controversy over health inequality and its causes did not, of course, spring into being *de novo* with the responses of Tory politicians to the work of Peter Townsend and his collaborators. But it has not, we believe, been pointed out quite what a long and full career remarks of the sort we have just quoted from Currie have had in twentieth-century British politics.[5]

Thus, the first task of this chapter is the relatively modest one of providing a historical framework within which to locate a contemporary issue in the sociology of health and illness. But the identification of long-term patterns within the history of the discourses of health and inequality is also very suggestive from a theoretical point of view. When we find Establishment spokespersons in the 1980s, the 1930s, and even the 1900s, all employing very similar debating repertoires, we are entitled to ask how and why such patterns of discourse have been sustained. Of course, what we are describing is, at one level, simply the career of a piece of political (and medical) rhetoric. But it is also, we think, something more.

We will attempt to argue that the association of ignorance with ill health is both a structured ideological response to the social threats and dangers posed by class inequality and a feature of the general pattern of control and discipline imposed upon the body in an advanced industrial society. In other words, Mrs Currie was, in her own way, stimulating the scrutiny of the status of the body within social theory with which all sociologists, post Bryan Turner, must now be concerned. She was displaying that the discourse of diet had not, in the late twentieth century, lost its moral dimension.

Health and ignorance past

In March 1936, Sir John Boyd Orr, Director of the Rowett Agricultural Research Institute in Aberdeen, published a study of the diet of the British population. He closed a chapter entitled 'Distribution of national income and food expenditure at different income levels' with the remark that:

> In group I, [the poorest group] … total food consumption is low and includes mainly cheap suppliers of energy and therefore cheap satisfiers of hunger, e.g. bread, potatoes and margarine. The consumption of more expensive foodstuffs … rises progressively with income … (Orr 1936:30).

Boyd Orr concluded that the diet of the poorest group, numbering 4.5 million people, was 'deficient in every nutrient examined', and that of the next poorest, numbering 9 million, was 'deficient in all the vitamins and minerals considered', (Orr 1936:49). Boyd Orr's methods of data collection, analysis, and presentation of his results, as well as the title of the book, *Food, Health and Income: Report on a Survey of Diet in Relation to Income*, all pointed towards the conclusion that it was income, or lack of income, which was likely to be the key factor in determining whether or not people obtained a healthy diet. The income of the poorer sections of the population was not sufficient to enable them to purchase adequate quantities of nourishing food.

Boyd Orr's conclusion that the income of a significant proportion of the population was inadequate to sustain health had also been arrived at by M'Gonigle and Kirby whose book, *Poverty and Public Health*, was also published in 1936. M'Gonigle was the Medical Officer of Health for Stockton-on-Tees. Earlier in the thirties other commentators, notably Allen Hutt (1933), had made similar arguments. In July 1936, in response to great public controversy, which had reached a new intensity with the appearance of *Food, Health and Income*, the House of Commons debated the issue of malnutrition among the working class, especially the unemployed and the low paid. Sir Kingsley Wood, the Minister of Health, replied to Labour's criticism of the government's welfare provisions by noting the lack of scientific unanimity as to the existence and causes of malnutrition:

> We often hear Sir John Orr quoted rather incompletely, but there is another equally eminent member of the Ministry of Health Committee, who can, I suppose, be equally regarded as an authority, and that is Professor Cathcart. He says that malnutrition is due not so much to poverty as to ignorance and other causes of the same kind ... (*Parliamentary Debates (Commons)* 1935–6).

The problems the poor experienced in nutrition were thus, so the official ministerial line went, to a large extent of their own making. Ignorance, it should be noted, frequently had in this rhetoric the status of a moral weakness. The government was not failing the poor; the poor were failing themselves.

When looking back upon this pre-war controversy over health inequality and its causes, it is not difficult to see M'Gonigle and Boyd Orr as occupying positions roughly equivalent to those of Townsend and Black in the 1980s, with Edwina Currie as a latter-day Kingsley Wood.[6] Kingsley Wood's remarks were part of a carefully prepared government response to an Opposition motion, whereas Currie's were made off-the-cuff to a reporter and earned her the disapproval of some members of her own party.[7] In the months that followed, however, Currie developed and refined her position. The notion that the health problems of the poor were largely a matter of ignorance and other individualistic shortcomings remained a central feature of her rhetoric – even if she expressed herself more sensitively, save on one or two other famous occasions.

Kingsley Wood was, moreover, not the first, as he would not be the last, Establishment figure to point to ignorance or some other moral failing as the root cause of the health problems of the lower orders. During the early Victorian period, the focus of attention of the sanitary reformers was upon housing, water supply and drains (Lewis 1952; Wohl 1983; Williams 1987) but in the latter part of the nineteenth century, with the introduction of compulsory education and the appointment of medical officers of health, a number of professional agencies began to take a more or less systematic interest in the home life and diet of the poor (Petty 1987:26–7; Tomes 1990). At the same time, many voluntary societies were founded with the specific aim of improving the domestic habits of the lower orders. Nearly every town had its Ladies Sanitary Committee, whose middle-class members visited the homes of the poor, attempting to influence child rearing and other household practices (Dwork 1987:125–6). The National Health Society, which was formed in 1872, sought, among other things, to encourage the teaching of hygiene and needlework in schools. They also produced handbills and other publications on health matters for the working class (Anon 1879). Several organizations, such as the Destitute Childrens Dinner Society, were particularly interested in the feeding of schoolchildren (Gilbert 1966:104). But the Society for Organising Charitable Relief and Repressing Mendacity (later to become the Charity Organisation Society) was concerned to ensure that school feeding gave no encouragement to parents to rely upon hand-outs (Mowat 1961:75).

At the turn of the century, complaints about the inadequate physique of potential recruits to the military led to official investigations into the extent of the problem of poor health among the working class. In Scotland, a Royal Commission on Physical Training was appointed in 1902. Mr Hugh Muir, Headmaster of Dobbies Loan School, in a very poor area of Glasgow, gave evidence to the Commission that the housewives in his area fed their families on 'Dry bread and tea mostly, no oatmeal or vegetables or soups of any description. The majority of them would not be troubled cooking dinner …'. When the chairman asked whether the 'old custom of a little oatmeal in a basin and a little hot water poured over it' had 'gone out', Muir replied 'Yes, they would not be troubled with it … the easier way is to go to the shop and get a loaf and tea …' (Royal Commission on Physical Training 1903:**2**, 584). Similarly, R.W. Bruce, Medical Officer to the Glasgow School Board, commented:

> A meal that is easily cooked, though it is of low food value, is preferred to one of richer nourishment, which takes time to prepare or trouble to cook. It is largely from that cause that porridge, broth and potatoes have disappeared from the meals of the poor … (Royal Commission on Physical Training 1903:**2**, 592).

Over a third of the 137 witnesses heard by the Commission had something substantial to say on the subject of the diet of the working class. Some pointed out that physical training would not improve the physique of underfed children. For example W.L. Mackenzie, Medical Inspector of the Local Government Board of Scotland, was of the opinion that 'More drill, with the same food, would be … hurtful in the highest degree' (Royal Commission on Physical Training 1903:**2**, 268). The Commission's Report accordingly recommended that School Boards should 'provide facilities for the provision of suitable food by voluntary agencies …' but should this '… prove inadequate … powers should be given to provide a meal, and to demand from parents a payment to meet the cost price' (Royal Commission on Physical Training 1903:**1**, 37).

In England, the publicity given from 1901 onwards to the high rejection rates of volunteers for the Boer War, led to the appointment of the Interdepartmental Committee on Physical Deterioration. The Committee was required to determine the causes of impaired physical development and how the physique and health of the people might be monitored and improved. Evidence was heard from medical witnesses and educationalists, and from representatives of the voluntary health groups referred to earlier.

Some of the voluntary health workers who appeared before the Committee had obviously been profoundly shocked by their experiences. One rather atypical visitor to working-class homes was Mrs Elliner Close who, by her own account, had spent many years travelling in England and abroad. Her attitudes were, however, very similar to those of the less adventurous visitors, whose habit it was to cross from their leafy suburbs to the local slums. Mrs Close told the Committee that 40 years earlier, when she lived among poor people in Scotland and Cheshire, 'the cooking was first rate'. Now, however:

> the girls ... have no sort of sense of duty; not the slightest. It is only amusement and pleasure with them. The last thing they think of is duty, and therefore, they do not trouble to cook or get up in the morning, and the children go to school without breakfast, because the woman is too idle to get up ... she is utterly indifferent ... (Interdepartmental Committee 1904:**2**, 115).

One of Mrs Close's worst experiences had been in Windsor where the bed was so filthy she had had to sleep on the floor and the food was uneatable. Apparently, the only thing that the housewives who lived in such places could think of was going to the theatre in London.

A number of the witnesses complained that the poor were inclined to spend their meagre resources in fish and chip shops or on tinned food. For example, Dr Robert Jones commented:

> The main point lies in education, especially of women, who should be taught how to choose and cook proper food ... I have visited places in remote country districts as well as in congested metropolitan areas and I have seen provision shops retailing tinned rabbits, tinned fish, tinned milk and even tinned 'madeira' and other cakes, most of which could be served fresh and clean locally by the house-wives (Interdepartmental Committee 1904:**2**, 398).

In general, the Committee's witnesses stressed ignorance and degenerate habits as causes of ill-health and inferior physique among the poor, much more strongly than poverty *per se*.

The Report of the Interdepartmental Committee, published in July 1904, recommended improvements in environmental health, curbs on juvenile smoking and adult drinking, encouragement of physical training, the inspection of schoolchildren and the provision of school meals. Domestic education for working-class girls was, however, presented as the best long-term solution to the nutritional problems of the poor. This last recommendation proved to be relatively uncontentious and gave a significant boost to the development of domestic science in Britain. Soon after the report appeared, the first female inspectors of schools were appointed and their investigations during 1905 and 1906 lead to the publication by the Board of Education of a *Special Report on the Teaching of Cookery to Public Elementary School Children* (Lawrence 1907). A few years later the Household and Social Science Department of Kings College for Women, (later Queen Elizabeth College), was established.

In contrast to the broad consensus of agreement that seems to have surrounded the need for domestic education, the proposal that the state should support school feeding resulted in prolonged and sometimes acrimonious controversy. The Scottish Royal Commission had admitted that the proposal to give School Boards the power to provide meals:

> raises serious questions. It is a matter for grave consideration whether the valuable asset to the nation of improved moral and physical state of a large number of future citizens counterbalances the evils of impaired parental responsibility ... We have no desire to give encouragement to any inclination of the parent to abandon any of his duties and responsibilities in regard to the feeding and clothing of children ... (Royal Commission on Physical Training 1903:**1**, 30).

In other words, because the problem of ill-health among the poor was conceived of in terms of moral, rather than economic, incapacity, it was thought likely that any supportive intervention would itself have dangerous moral consequences.

The pros and cons of providing school meals were extensively debated in parliament, in medical circles, and in the press. The government employed the delaying tactic of appointing, in March 1905, a further Interdepartmental Committee to investigate existing provision and to report whether school feeding could be 'better organised without any charge upon public funds' (Interdepartmental Committee 1905:**1**, vii). Several of the witnesses to this Committee sternly warned about the possible harmful effects of state-supported school feeding. Miss M. Dendy, Member of the Manchester Education Committee and Vice Chairman of the Sub-Committee for Feeding Destitute Children, commented:

> Home conditions are at the root of the bodily suffering of children. Improper food taken at irregular hours, lack of sleep and dirt have all done irreparable damage before the child is three years old. To these may be added great indulgence and lack of discipline. Any agency for helping children which relieves the parents of responsibility must make the children's condition worse (Interdepartmental Committee 1905:**2**, 206).

She recommended the criminal prosecution of fathers as an encouragement for them to feed their children properly.

In the first two decades of the century, one of the most vociferous supporters of school feeding, in particular, and the increased involvement of the state in welfare provision in general, was L.G. Chiozza Money, a Liberal MP and the author of the influential book, *Riches and Poverty* (1905). He firmly rejected the arguments that state support for school feeding would have a detrimental effect upon family life:

> The chief deterrent to many is fear that parents will be demoralised by free meals at the schools. It must be realised by those who entertain this fear that the parents are often already thoroughly demoralised, and that their demoralisation in the greatest majority of cases has resulted from the conditions imposed upon them by our social system. They are what they are because of circumstances over which their control was nominal (Money 1905:181).

But even Chiozza Money conceded that a 'large proportion' of housewives were ignorant as well as necessitous, 'lacking both the means to feed themselves and their children properly, and the training to apply the means if they had them'. He therefore urged that:

> Girls should not leave school ... until they have been seriously trained in domestic duties. At present we herd them in classes of 60 or 80, and leave a teacher, herself often ignorant of the chief duties of womanhood, to impart to them a smattering of secondary importance. Able to write badly, to cipher inaccurately, and to read a novelette, the girl goes forth from the school 'educated', and more ignorant of the essential things than the untutored savage (Money 1906:166–7).

Thus, it should be noted that, at this time, even those who denied that the state provision of school meals would be demoralizing were still prepared to conceive of the problem of faulty feeding in the home as having its roots, at least partly, in the individual moral shortcomings of parents, especially mothers.

The consensus of opinion as to the moral causes of ill-feeding represented by the Royal Commission and the Interdepartmental Committees was also voiced by the health establishment. During the early part of the twentieth century, one of the most powerful figures in the field of public health within the apparatus of the state was Sir George Newman. He was Chief Medical Officer to the Board of Education from 1907 and Chief Medical Officer at the Ministry of Health, from 1919. He was the first incumbent of these two positions, both of which he held until 1935. In examining the position of the state within this discourse on diet, health, ignorance and income, the writings of Sir George Newman are a good place to start.

Newman consistently emphasized the importance of ignorance as a cause of health problems. In 1906, for example, in his book *Infant Mortality: A*

Social Problem, he asserted 'it is ignorance and carelessness of mothers that directly causes a large proportion of infant mortality' (Newman 1906:221). What was needed, he argued, was 'training in those arts of domestic management of which compulsory education has deprived the girls of the artisan classes' (Newman 1906:268). In 1907, the year in which he became Chief Medical Officer at the Board of Education, Newman published another book, entitled *The Health of the State*, in which he remarked:

> money paid for food, is unfortunately, often spent very wastefully, in response to silly advertisements or because of ignorance, and among the necessary reforms in the domestic life of the people at the present time, not the least important is food reform – the money laid out upon, and the selection of food (Newman 1907:34).

Newman was soon expressing these views in official publications. In his annual report to the Board of Education for 1910, for example, he summarized a very long document by concluding that the useful role which could be played by governmental agencies was very limited:

> At the best ... the work which the Local Education Authorities can do in directly preventing and remedying the evils of malnutrition has somewhat definite limits. The proper and sufficient feeding of children is primarily a function of the home, and it is to the gradual improvement of the home that Local Education Authorities must primarily look for relief from the special difficulties which confront them through the malnutrition of the child (Newman 1911:258).

Thereafter, he regularly devoted a portion of his annual report to encouraging Local Education Authorities to devise schemes for the domestic education of housewives. In this section of his report for 1914, he commented:

> The three causes of malnutrition in children are poverty, ignorance and the neglect of their parents, and the greatest of these is probably ignorance. Malnutrition is frequently the result not of lack of food, but improper food, and it is found in homes where wages are good (Newman 1915:220).

In 1920, in an address to the National Health Society, Newman noted that, since people in Britain received a 'living wage' and there existed 'a sufficient yield of ... food necessary to ... health', therefore if people did 'not live the healthy life' it must be because they lacked the relevant knowledge (Newman 1920:13).

However, only a limited part of the responsibility for educating ignorant people lay with the state – as he explained in 1925, 'In every direction the prevention of disease is becoming a personal concern rather than exclusively a matter dependent upon the central, or even the local, authorities responsible for the supervision of Public Health' (Newman 1925:4). Newman here ascribed a key role to voluntary organizations:

> However excellent the propaganda undertaken by the Local Authorities and other governmental bodies, there would still remain an immense field for voluntary effort ... The character and tradition of the people of Great Britain are such that they will elect, and rightly, to be arbiters of their own fate. They will not accept that which is foisted upon them against their will (Newman 1925:17).

Newman's opinion as to the relationship, or rather the lack of a relationship, between income and nutrition remained essentially unmodified throughout his career. In his memoir, *The Building of a Nation's Health*, published in 1939, he commented that:

> to assess the nutrition of a whole nation only on estimates of family income, or only on estimates of money expended out of family income on food per family, or only on estimates of the amount and character of food purchased per family, is likely to prove fallacious (Newman 1939:354).

In what was obviously a response to the work of Boyd Orr and other critics, Newman firmly endorsed the conclusion arrived at by the Interdepartmental Committee on Physical Deterioration, 35 years earlier, 'There is no relation between the total earnings of a householder, and the quantity or quality of the food going into the household' (Newman 1939:354).

There are two points which it is important to note concerning the views we just have attributed to George Newman. The first is that the emphasis on ignorance and moral failings as the cause of health and nutrition problems was a central element in Newman's arguments against proposed extensions of the state's existing activities in the field of health that did not meet with his approval, or the approval of his political masters. Because the real reasons for poor nutrition and other health problems were moral and individualistic, rather than economic, government intervention might do more harm than good. It might sap the energies of self-help, undermine the principled independence of the sturdy yeomen and women of England. Secondly, when Newman pronounced on these issues he spoke not merely as a high-ranking government official, but also as a doctor and a scientist. He cloaked himself and his opinions in the full authority of contemporary medical science.

And, it must be conceded, Newman's position was eminently defensible in the terms of the scientific opinion of his day. Perhaps Newman himself was really more of a civil servant than a scientist, but there were plenty of working research scientists who would undoubtedly have fully endorsed his pronouncements. Consider, for example, the opinions of Noël Paton,

Regius Professor of Physiology at Glasgow University. In 1913, Paton supervised a survey of diet and dietary habit among the Glasgow working class. The report of this survey concluded that many poorer people were inadequately fed but it was felt that all but those in penury:

> ought to be able to afford enough to eat. Where the diet is notably inadequate, this is due mostly to bad marketing [that is, bad buying of food] and to waste, and also to ignorance as to the best kind of food to buy (Lindsay 1913:12).

The Glasgow report was very positively reviewed in the *British Medical Journal*, which endorsed its conclusion that 'proper school training in cooking and marketing' was 'the best corrective' (Anon 1913:674–675).

In 1917, very similar views were expressed by Paton's colleague, Dr Leonard Findlay, who would shortly become Glasgow University's Professor of Medical Paediatrics. In a paper entitled 'Causes of infantile mortality' published as part of an MRC Report, Findlay cast doubt upon the efficacy of Milk Depots and 'Infant Cliniques'. (Glasgow Corporation had opened its first milk depot in 1904.) He also strongly controverted the view that low wage levels contributed to the high infant death rate. The real cause of infant mortality lay, he argued, in poor hygiene. He acknowledged the benefits of slum clearance but continued, 'It must be admitted that ignorance on the part of the parents may play a certain part ...' (Findlay 1917:41).

Paton and Findlay's views on the origins of poor nutrition and physique were most highly developed in their joint MRC report on 'Poverty, Nutrition and Growth' (Paton and Findlay 1926). Using quantitative means of assessing 'maternal efficiency', 'poverty', 'under-feeding' and 'over-crowding', they concluded that, of these, 'maternal efficiency' was the factor most closely associated with variations in the condition of the child. They also concluded that 'maternal efficiency' was not 'directly and immediately associated with poverty'. It was acknowledged that impaired 'maternal efficiency' was, to an extent, associated with bad housing, but Paton and Findlay did not conclude from this that the problems associated with maternal inefficiency should be addressed by raising economic status:

> What is not demonstrated is that simple increase of income would be followed by improvement in the condition of the children. Bad parents, irrespective of their incomes, tend to select bad houses, as the money is often spent on other things. The saying that 'what is wrong with the poor is their poverty' is not substantiated by these investigations ... (Paton and Findlay 1926:305).

Similar sentiments were expressed by another Glaswegian scientist, the chemical physiologist Professor Edward Cathcart. Like Paton and Findlay, Cathcart continually stressed the role of character as a major determinant of the health of working-class families, strongly endorsing the conclusions of his colleagues as to the importance of 'maternal efficiency'. Cathcart acknowledged that a section of the population was inadequately fed. However, the fault did not lie with inadequate income, but with what he described as the 'much deeper' causes of 'bad buying and bad cooking' (Cathcart 1931:178). The solution, he said, lay in education. Lessons in cooking, given as part of the school curriculum, should be adapted to the circumstances of the working-class housewife and be based upon 'one-pot, one small gas-ring' facilities. Cathcart supported the local domestic science college and approved of the staging, by voluntary groups, of economical cookery demonstrations in working-class areas (Smith 1986:96–8, 319–20).

As we have seen, it was to the work of Cathcart that Sir Kingsley Wood, the Minister of Health, chose to turn for support when responding to Opposition claims that the income of the poorer sections of the population was not adequate to maintain health. It is worth mentioning that Cathcart was well aware of the political implications of his views on nutrition. In 1931 he had privately warned officials in the Ministry of Health that an advisory committee's report setting out principles of good dietary practice for Medical Officers in charge of institutions (Ministry of Health 1932) could have political repercussions. Sir George Newman received a memorandum which reported that:

> the diet recommended ... is something much better than the average working man can afford, and he [Cathcart] is afraid that if it is embodied in an official document it may be seized upon by transitional beneficiaries and others as a yard stick to measure what their allowances should be (Carnwarth 1931).

It is therefore unlikely that Cathcart would have been adverse to Wood quoting him in defence of government policy in the context of the 1936 debate.

Throughout the 1930s, the issue of how active a role the state could and should play in the promotion of the nation's health and welfare was very actively debated. Reformers such as Boyd Orr and M'Gonigle, together with pressure groups such as the Committee against Malnutrition and the Children's Minimum Committee, called for the introduction of a cheap food policy and/or the provision of improved monetary and material benefits (Webster 1982; 1985). Other scientists and scientific spokespersons urged the state to take more responsibility for the feeding of the nation in the name of scientific efficiency (Smith 1986; Petty 1987). For example, Walter Fletcher and Edward Mellanby, successive Secretaries of the MRC, sought to persuade the government to promote feeding along proper scientific principles, as revealed by the new knowledge of the importance of vitamins and minerals in the diet. Their approach to the nation's health problems might be termed 'scientific statism'. In essence, they wanted the results of the nutrition research which had been funded by the MRC to be incorporated within government policy. Mellanby argued for the establishment of a Board of Nutrition which would coordinate research into nutrition and would guide the Ministry of Health in assuming greater control over institutional feeding. Mellanby also noted the 'large trade carried on by cookshops in poorer areas', but rather than condemning this as an example of the ignorance and degeneracy of the working class, he saw it as providing an example for the state to emulate. He suggested the 'setting up of public and official organisations whereby people can obtain food already prepared for consumption either at home or on the premises' (Mellanby 1927:636). Needless to say, such a suggestions was anathema to Cathcart and others of his voluntarist persuasion.

Throughout the 1930s, ministers and civil servants were, in contrast to the social and scientific reformers, anxious to minimize public expenditure. Their preferred alternative remedy of health education had the advantage of being relatively cheap, especially if undertaken largely by voluntary agencies. However, the onset of war in 1939 saw the establishment of the Ministry of Food and a radical revision of health policy. A system of food rationing was introduced, devised along scientific principles and with special provisions for children and for pregnant and nursing women. Fortification of margarine with vitamin D was introduced and state-run 'British Restaurants' were established (Hammond 1956:381–412). The welfare foods scheme was started in 1941, providing cheap, and eventually free, orange juice, cod liver oil and vitamin tablets. In many respects therefore the wartime food provisions embodied many of the proposals made, in the pre-war period, by the 'scientific statists'.

It should however be remembered that wartime was also a heyday of voluntarism.[8] Great emphasis was placed upon the education of the public in nutritional and culinary matters. The Food Leaders Scheme, for example, created a network of volunteers to undertake a programme of demonstrations of economical cooking – thus implementing a policy which had long been advocated by Cathcart. By 1945, there were 15,000 Food Leaders, (Clark 1945:75–8). Thus, in many respects, the World War II food programme harmoniously combined the statist and voluntarist approaches to health policy. This was not, however, to last. In 1944, Cathcart raised the issue of the proper and appropriate role of the state *vis-à-vis* the individual in the health sphere, in the context of a contribution to the discussion on post-war reconstruction. In what was virtually the opening salvo of a renewed debate between the voluntarist and the statist approaches, he wrote:

> A great deal has been written about the present day short-comings ... in connection with the preservation of health, mental and physical, of the people ... The suggestion is that the powers-that-be have been laggard in taking cogniz-

ance of the urgent need of improving the lot of the lower paid members of the community (Cathcart 1944:3).

But, he continued, the existence of health 'black spots' was not always to be:

> ascribed to dilatoriness on the part of the authorities. The people themselves have to share the blame. Many are careless, indifferent and ignorant. They do not realise, to take a simple example, the many dangers to communal health of environmental and personal lack of cleanliness (Cathcart 1944:3).

Shades again of Mrs Currie – especially when we note that Cathcart associated his moralistic position on health matters with a general statement of robust political individualism:

> The popular word today is planning. It is altogether too popular and it is dangerous ... A world run on strictly bureaucratic lines or scientific basis could be guaranteed to destroy initiative. Petty officialdom is anti-pathetic to the British way of life, living and growth and the spirit of service (Cathcart 1944:48).

Health and ignorance present

If we return to our own era, during the Thatcher years, large-scale public controversy over social health issues was probably first occasioned by the appearance of the *Report on Inequalities in Health related to Social Class*, the Black Report, in August 1980. Like Boyd Orr's *Food, Health and Income*, in the 1930s, the Black Report quickly became a bible for the Opposition and for health agencies critical of the government. Mr Patrick Jenkin, Secretary of State for Health and Social Security, wrote a dismissive preface to the publication and then maintained a virtual silence for six months. When he finally went on the offensive, this is what he said:

> It may be that there is a correlation between socio-economic group and state of health. But Black has not been able to identify causes which indicate specific treatment ... On the other hand, it does appear there is a very definite correlation between education and better health ... All the evidence about illness from smoking has had a dramatic effect on better educated people, but has had virtually no effect on the less well educated. Now is that class-oriented or is it education-oriented? (quoted in Deitch 1981:736).

The manner in which Jenkin referred to smoking marks these comments as a product of the later twentieth century but much else of what he said will now be familiar to the reader.

Jenkin's rhetoric was that of the government as a whole. In July 1981, Sir George Young, Under-Secretary of State for Health, replied to a Labour question which drew attention to the Black Report in the following manner 'I see the progress being made by encouraging health education, personal responsibility for health, and encouraging voluntary organisations to help ...' (quoted in Anon 1981).

During the months and years following the publication of the report, many of the arguments formulated by those who wanted to resist its conclusions would not have been out of place as contributions to the *Food, Health and Income* debate of 50 years earlier, or even as evidence to the Interdepartmental Committee on Physical Deterioration, nearly 80 years previously. For example, in May 1983 Dr D.L. Crombie, Director of the Birmingham Research Unit of the Royal College of General Practitioners, gave a keynote lecture entitled 'Social Class and Health Status, Inequality or Difference?' which amounted to a direct response to the Black Report. In Crombie's view:

> The main distinguishing features between social classes is the relative capacity to cope, to deal with life's problems in general ... This ability to cope is probably determined partly genetically and partly by formal education, family upbringing and cultural influence ... if a relative ability to cope is the distinguishing feature, educational influences in their widest sense are likely to have more effect than simple increases in spendable cash (Crombie 1984:13).

Whether or not he was aware of the historical resonances of his words, it is evident that Crombie was re-stating, albeit in a somewhat different vocabulary, with a slightly different nuance, the old individualistic, moralistic explanation of the existence of inequalities in health. Such inequalities were not the fault of socio-economic circumstances, he argued; they were principally the fault of the people themselves. Like Newman, Paton, Findlay and Cathcart before him, Crombie concluded that education was the best answer.

Crombie made his remarks in response, it should be noted, to the uncompromising stress which the authors of the Black Report had put upon what they called the 'materialist structuralist' explanation of health inequality. They, like Boyd Orr, M'Gonigle and the Committee Against Malnutrition, saw class inequalities in income as the root cause of excessive ill-health in the lower social classes. Only if the problem of poverty was addressed, if some degree of economic adjustment took place, could the problem of health inequality be reduced.

The aim of Mrs Thatcher's government re-shuffle in September 1986, in which Edwina Currie became Junior Health Minister, was to strengthen the DHSS team in order to counter the Labour Party's propaganda offensive on health issues. According to her book *Life Lines* (1989), when Currie arrived at the Department of Health, the first thing she did was to write a paper entitled 'The Conservatives and the NHS – Moving the Goalposts'. She explained that 'The objective ... was to develop themes incorporating the Conservative philosophies of personal responsibility [and] a diminished role for the State' (Currie 1989:5). A week after writing this paper she made her famous, or perhaps notorious, visit to Newcastle.

By 1989, Mrs Currie had had time to formulate her criticisms more carefully:

> The statistics that were thrust under my nose in Newcastle had demonstrated ... that life expectancy could be as much as ten years less in one city ward ... than in a neighbouring ward across the river. ... What annoyed me about such surveys is that they went on to measure indices of deprivation, but not of smoking; levels of poverty, but not of heavy drinking and alcoholism; amounts available to spend on food, but not what actually went into the shopping basket ... They could tell us how many houses had no inside toilet ... but they could not tell us how many heads were empty of the basic information needed to feed the family a sensible diet on that restricted budget (Currie 1989:25).

She claimed that during her period in office the objective of 'moving the goalposts' had indeed been accomplished. Within the Department of Health, the goals of the prevention of disease and the promotion of good health were now increasingly being pursued by means of encouraging people to change their life-styles and by emphasizing the need to accept personal responsibility. This programme fitted in, Currie said, with her own belief 'that the state was not and should not be all-powerful' (Currie 1989:245). 'Moving the goalposts' at the Department of Health was, she said, an expression of the 'essence of the Thatcher revolution' (Currie 1989:241) – 'people were ready to take more responsibility in a host of ways' (Currie 1989:249). One of the ironies of the story of the rhetorical connection between health and ignorance is that Currie self-consciously presented her analysis of the nation's health problems as new and revolutionary – as a bold escape from the older, tired political certainties of collectivism. But any one who has read Sir George Newman or Professor Edward Cathcart is entitled to a distinct feeling of *déjà vu*. We hope that, in this chapter, we have shown that in fact Currie was enunciating what her erstwhile political mistress would no doubt have termed 'Victorian values'.

Discussion

One obvious explanation for the regularity with which ill-health has been attributed to ignorance is that such an argument directly serves economic interests. If the problems the working class and the poor experience in nutrition are, to a large extent, of their own making, then increased monetary investment in health care or social security, or the instituting of a cheap food policy, would not be an effective means of alleviating the problems caused by inadequate nutrition. The government need not therefore acknowledge any great degree of responsibility for the situation and a policy of minimal intervention in the health sphere is thereby legitimated. The preferred solution, health education, has, of course, the advantage of being relatively cheap and of not requiring structural economic change which might damage the social standing of the middle classes. Given the habitual concern of the Treasury to minimize the cost of health provision, any explanation of government rhetoric in terms of economic interest, narrowly conceived, is undoubtedly valid. It might be noted that the present authors stressed very similar considerations in an earlier paper (Smith and Nicolson 1989). This narrow economic interest explanation, moreover, resonates with comments made by Marxist analysts, such as Vincent Navarro (1976; 1978), concerning the ideological role of the state in debates over the cause and character of illness in contemporary capitalist society. There is a tendency, Navarro argues, for hegemonic class agencies to attempt systematically to obscure the structural and environmental causes of illness by emphasizing individualistic factors, especially moral failings, as the causes of ill-health, thus deflecting attention and blame from the material circumstances of labour. This chapter may thus be seen as an attempt to provide some much needed historical and empirical flesh for the notoriously bare theoretical bones of Navarro's political–economic analysis.

However, there are elements of the twentieth-century debate surrounding health and ignorance which highlight the need to elaborate upon the 'narrow economic interest' explanation, if a comprehensive understanding of recent diet and nutrition discourse is to be arrived at. It should be noted that middle-class surveillance of working-class eating habits was as much concerned with how they ate as what, or how much, food was consumed. The voluntary visitors commented adversely, not merely on the fact that the poor composed their meals mostly of bread and tea, but also that approved infant feeding rituals were not observed and that the older members of the family did not sit down all together to dine (Petty 1987:390).[9] In other words, concern with what the working classes put on their plates was only one aspect, albeit an important one, of a more general mapping-out of the behavioural differences between the lower and middle classes. No doubt such differentiation, and its moral overtones, had its ultimate basis in the material circumstances of the class structure. No doubt Navarro is right that the ascription of moral blame had strategic utility for the hegemonic class. But any argument so based on narrow economic interest cannot, by itself, explain why particular aspects of working-class behaviour were chosen for middle-class moral disapprobation.

What seems to have happened was that the voluntary and professional critics of the working class commented most adversely upon those aspects of working-class behaviour that seemed the most significantly and threatenly different from the self-conscious middle-class ideal and its disciplines. But we must remember that middle-class behaviour had itself undergone significant changes during the nineteenth century. In an important recent study, Nancy Tomes (1990) has documented how, in the period between 1870 and 1900, the upper and middle classes became much more concerned with domestic hygiene and sanitation than they had previously been.[10] Overall, the late nineteenth century was characterized by the development of a cult of domesticity which invested family life, and especially child-rearing, with enormous social, moral and medical significance (Donzelot 1979; Lewis 1980).

It was, in other words, against a background of their own domestic behaviour that the middle classes sought to discipline and transform the household arrangements of the working class. Thus, while it may be true that the ascription of moral blame to the working class is in the 'objective' economic interests of the hegemonic class, the particular form such moral blaming takes at any particular time must be seen as being dependent upon the particular cultural circumstances of upper- and middle-class life at that time. It follows from this that, before we can arrive at a full understanding of the dietary rhetoric employed by the hegemonic class against the working class, we must comprehend the significance given by the hegemonic class to food and nutrition within its own domestic arrangements. We must, in other words, marry an anthropological perspective on food and the body to political–economic analyses.

It is perhaps appropriate here to pause and consider that it is only recently that the sociology of health and illness has turned its attention to food, diet and nutrition (Murcott 1983; Calnan 1990). Accordingly we are, it is probably fair to say, still a little short of theoretical sophistication in this area. Nor have we fully got to grips with its empirical complexity. This comparative neglect is, of course, regrettable, not least because it entails that the historical importance of ideas about diet and food has not yet been fully explored or appreciated. It is arguable that, as Foucault has maintained, a rationalizing and disciplining discourse about diet developed and flourished long before similar discourses concerning sexuality, time, work, rationality or whatever. The works of the Greek physicians, for example, devote hundreds of pages to dietary advice, while relatively little is said about the management of sexuality. Likewise, the discipline imposed within monastic institutions, which Foucault takes as the model and the precursor of the disciplines of the asylum, the prison and the factory, was, he put it, about 'food, food, food' (Foucault 1984:340).

One of the few theorists to have given serious attention to the issues of food and nutrition is Bryan Turner (1982a; 1982b; 1987). Following Foucault (1979), Turner sees the regulation of diet as 'a part of a broader regimen for the government of the body', as part, in other words, of the reckoning and controlling of the body by the systematic application of power and knowledge (Turner 1987:22). Even in the sixteenth century, solutions for social disorder were sought in the cultivation of regular and sober lifestyles among the population. Dietary restrictions formed part of this early modern bodily discipline, at least as far as the upper and middle classes were concerned. During the late nineteenth century, Turner writes, this older medical and religious discourse on diet was transformed into a new, secular science. The scientific analysis of nutrition was motivated by concerns to improve the efficiency and cost-effectiveness of farms, penal institutions, factories, armies and so on. Social and dietary surveys of the working class were undertaken both to counteract the social and political threats apparently posed by an unhealthy and disaffected working class and as integral aspects of a systematic programme for the bureaucratic and rationalizing management of manpower and production. In several respects, Turner's treatment of diet closely parallels E.P. Thompson's (1967) classic account of how time was rationalized and transformed by the imposition of rigorous shift discipline upon the factory workforce.

It will be apparent that the empirical story we have presented above supports Turner's thesis in several respects. Turner presents the medical disciplinary discourse of diet as having been first applied within the behaviour of the middle class and only secondarily extended to bring it to bear upon the urban working class. While some of the details of his historical description of this process have, we think rightly, been challenged (Aronson 1984; Turner 1985), the overall principle would appear to be a sound one. The discipline of diet would seem, in this respect, to mirror the discipline of domestic cleanliness – taken up by the middle class in the nineteenth century, used as a benchmark to expose the inadequacies of the working class in the late nineteenth and twentieth. One might also draw a parallel here with physical training, the discourse of which is, as we have seen, often closely related to that of diet. The first group to be subjected to a systematic discipline of physical training, outside of the armed forces, were the male schoolchildren of the middle and professional classes (Haley 1978). While the investigation of the social history of the body along these lines is only just beginning, it seems likely that its conclusions will be just those that a reader of Foucault (1980) would have predicted – the first objects upon which power exercises its creative effects are the powerful.

There is one respect, however, in which our account differs, at least in nuance, from Turner's. Turner notes that, in his account of the development of the social control of the body, Foucault describes both the rationalization of external physical control and the cultivation of the 'inner discipline of private conscience' (Turner 1982b:23). Likewise, Turner draws upon the work of those authors, such as Navarro, who have emphasized the ideological importance of discourses which invoke moral individualism and personal responsibility. But in his own description of the development of dietary discipline in the twentieth century, Turner stresses panoptical surveillance and scientific management, and does not place any weight upon the moral dimension of the disciplinary discourse. He writes:

> ... the new discourse of the body is shorn of its religious terminology. The body is no longer informed by 'divine Sobriety', but by calories and proteins so that discipline and efficiency can be measured with precision and certainty (Turner 1982b:29).

This line of argument is in marked contrast to his discussions of dietetics in the nineteenth and earlier centuries, in which he emphasizes the central importance of moral connotations.

As the evidence we have presented above makes clear, a moralizing dimension within dietary discourse continued to be important throughout the twentieth century, and continues to be important to the present day. Indeed there would seem to have been considerable tension, within the general project of maximizing the efficiency of the workforce, between those who urged the rigorous implementation of scientific knowledge, regardless of moral consideration, and those who sought to combine surveillance with moral disapprobation. On the one hand, there were commentators who, like Fletcher and Mellanby, wished to employ sweeping state intervention to rationalize the diet of the working class along the lines of the newer knowledge of nutrition. On the other hand, there were those who, like Newman, Cathcart and Currie, sought to effect changes in working-class behaviour by moral suasion and example. While one group may be seen as seeking to extend, in exactly the manner described by Turner, the modes of efficient institutional feeding to the population as a whole, the other vigorously opposed such a programme, precisely because they feared it would compromise the development of the 'inner discipline of private conscience'. It is probably fair to say that, at least in Britain, the latter group was, over the twentieth century as a whole, at least as important as the former, as far as the rhetoric of public policy-making was concerned.

Therefore, it must be concluded that the new secular discourse of diet, while undoubtedly drawing much of its content and inspiration from a programme of scientific rationalization, cannot be understood as being formed wholly or purely by a rationalizing agenda. At the very least, the rationalizing agenda must be understood, not as having its character wholly predetermined by the dynamics of class conflict or the extension of power relations, but also as being moulded and formed by intra-class conflicts and strategic differences, within particular historical and cultural contexts. The number of contradictory forces bearing upon the government of society ensures that the discourse of the government of the body displays a genuine and complex historical relativity. It would appear likely, moreover, that the body is too deeply imbued with moral significance for scientific rationalization, or considerations of efficiency, ever wholly to dominate how it will be conceived. Perhaps the empirical material presented above might lead us to the tentative conclusion that, while what the poor are supposed not to know may be a historical and social variable, to some people the poor have always been ignorant as to what is good for their bodies.

Acknowledgements

Earlier versions of this chapter were given to seminars in Glasgow and Amsterdam, as well as to the BSA Conference in Manchester. We would like to thank all those who provided us with comments, questions and criticisms, on these and other occasions, especially Stuart Blume, Alan Ducklin, Loet Leydesdorff, Debbie Kemer, Alesia Maltz, N.W. Pirie, Reginald Passmore, Gerard de Vries and J. Yudkin. During the preparation of this chapter, Drs Smith and Nicolson have been in receipt of financial support from the Wellcome Trust to whom we wish to record our gratitude.

Notes

1 Professor Townsend has been prominent in recent debates concerning social inequality in health, especially since the appearance of the Black Report, Black *et al.* (1980), of which he was one of the co-authors.
2 Quoted in 'Currie chides the unhealthy North' *The Times*, 24 September 1986, 1f.
3 About two weeks after her remarks in Newcastle, the television programme, *World in Action*, gave Currie the opportunity to expand upon her position. She was quoted in *The Times* as having commented: 'Every family could spend less on smoking and drinking, and switch that money to a better diet.' *The Times*, 6 October 1986, 2f.
4 For a review see S. Macintyre, (1986).
5 G. Jones (1986:162–3), A. Karpf (1988:35) and C. Petty (1989:fn 123) have all made passing remarks upon certain similarities between the health debates of the 1930s and 1980s.
6 The historical and geographical parallels between his position and that of M'Gonigle are evidently appreciated by Townsend himself; see the introduction to Townsend *et al.* (1988).
7 'Currie booed by delegates', *The Times*, 9 October 1986, 1b.
8 For an overview of the history of the voluntary movement in Britain, see Finlayson (1990).
9 For an extended discussion of the development of middle-class infant feeding practices in the late nineteenth century, see Lewis (1980).
10 Tomes (1990) concerns herself almost entirely with the USA but much of what she says is obviously relevant to the British context. We await a British study along similar lines.

References

Anon (1913), 'Diet of the labouring classes', *British Medical Journal*, **1**:674–5.

Anon (1981), 'News and notes. Inequalities in health', *British Medical Journal*, **283**:567.

Aronson, N. (1984), 'Comment on Bryan Turner's "The government of the body: medical regimens and the rationalisation of diet"', *British Journal of Sociology*, **35**:62–5.

Black, D., Morris, J.N., Smith, C. and Townsend, P. (1980), *Inequalities in Health. Report of a Research Working Group*, London: DHSS. Also published (1982) as *Inequalities in Health. The Black Report*, London: Pelican.

Calnan, M. (1990), 'Food and health: a comparison of beliefs and practices in middle-class and working-class households', in Cunningham-Burley, S. and McKeganey, N.P. (eds), *Readings in Medical Sociology*, London: Tavistock/Routledge.

Carnwarth, T. (1931), 'Memorandum' Carnwath to Newman 1/12/31, Public Records Office, Kew, MH 56/51.

Cathcart, E.P. (1931), 'The significance of dietary studies', *Journal of the Royal Sanitary Institute*, **52**:178–183.

Cathcart, E.P. (1944), *Communal Health*, The British Way Series No. 10, Glasgow: Glasgow University Press.

Clark, F. le Gros (1945), 'Food advice in the post-war world', *Health Education Journal*, **3**:75–8.

Crombie, D.L. (1984), *Social Class and Health Status Inequality or Difference? Fourth McConaghey Memorial Lecture (May 1983)*, Royal College of General Practitioners, Occasional Paper 25, Exeter: RCGP.

Currie, E. (1989), *Life Lines*, London: Sedgwick and Jackson.

Deitch, R. (1981), 'Commentary from Westminster, Mr Jenkin on the Black Report', *The Lancet*, **1**:735–6.

Donzelot, J. (1979), *The Policing of Families*, New York: Pantheon.

Dwork, D. (1987), *War is Good for Babies and other Young Children: A History of the Infant and Child Welfare Movement in England, 1898–1918*, London: Tavistock.

Findlay, L. (1917), 'The causes of infantile mortality', in *The Mortalities of Birth Infancy and Childhood*, Medical Research Committee Special Report Series 10, 37–42, London: HMSO.

Finlayson, G. (1990), 'A moving frontier: voluntarism and the state in British social welfare', *Twentieth Century British History*, **1**:183–206.

Foucault, M. (1984), 'On the genealogy of ethics: An overview of a work in progress', in Rabinow, P. (ed.), *The Foucault Reader*, New York: Random House.

Foucault, M. (1979), *Discipline and Punish: The Birth of the Prison*, Harmondsworth: Penguin.

Foucault, M. (1980), *Power/Knowledge. Selected Interviews and Other Writings 1972–77*, Gordon, C. (ed.), Brighton: Harvester Press.

Gilbert, B.B. (1966), *The Evolution of National Insurance in Great Britain: The Origins of the Welfare State*, London: Michael Joseph.

Haley, B. (1978), *The Healthy Body and Victorian Culture*, Cambridge, Massachusetts: Harvard University Press.
Hammond, R.J. (1956), *Food, Volume II, Studies in Administration and Control*, History of the Second World War United Kingdom Series, London: HMSO and Longmans, Green.
Hutt, A. (1933), *The Condition of the Working Class in Britain*, London: Maurice Laurence.
Interdepartmental Committee on Physical Deterioration (1904), *Report*, Vol. 1 Report and Appendix, Cd 2175 xxxii 1; Vol. 2 List of witnesses and evidence, Cd 2210 xxxii 145; Vol. 3 Appendix and index, Cd 2186 xxxii 655.
Interdepartmental Committee on Medical Inspection and Feeding of Children attending the Public Elementary Schools (1906), *Report*, Vol. 1 Report and Appendices, Cd 2779 xlvii 1; Vol. 2 List of witnesses, evidence, appendices and index. Cd 2784 xlvii 157.
Jones, G. (1986), *Social Hygiene in Twentieth Century Britain*, London: Croom Helm.
Karpf, A. (1988), *Doctoring the Media: The Reporting of Health and Medicine*, London: Routledge.
Lawrence, M.A. (1907), *Board of Education Special Report on the Teaching of Cookery to Public Elementary School Children in England and Wales*, London: HMSO.
Lewis, J. (1980), *The Politics of Motherhood*, London: Croom Helm.
Lewis, R.A. (1952), *Edwin Chadwick and the Public Health Movement 1832–1854*, London: Longmans, Green.
Lindsay, D.E. (1913), *Report upon the Study of the Diet of the Labouring Classes in the City of Glasgow carried out under the auspices of the Corporation of the City*, with Introduction by Professor D.N. Paton, Glasgow: Glasgow Corporation.
Macintyre, S. (1986), 'The patterning of health by social position in contemporary Britain: Directions for sociological research', *Social Science and Medicine*, **23**:393–415.
Mellanby, E. (1927), 'Duties of the state in relation to the nation's food supply', *British Medical Journal*, **2**:633–6.
Ministry of Health (1932), *Memorandum to the Minister on the Criticism and Improvement of Diets*, Advisory Committee on Nutrition, London: HMSO.
M'Gonigle, G.C.M. and Kirby, J. (1936), *Poverty and Public Health*, London: Victor Gollanz.
Money, L.G. Chiozza (1905), *Riches and Poverty*, London: Methuen.
Mowat, C.L. (1961), *The Charity Organisation Society 1869–1913. Its Ideas and Work*, London: Methuen.
Murcott, A. (1983), *The Sociology of Food and Eating*, Aldershot: Gower.
Navarro, V. (1976), *Medicine under Capitalism*, New York: Prodist.
Navarro, V. (1978), *Class Struggle, the State and Medicine: An Historical and Contemporary Analysis of the Medical Sector in Great Britain*, London: Martin Robertson.
Newman, G. (1906), *Infant Mortality: A Social Problem*, London: Methuen.
Newman, G. (1907), *The Health of the State*, Social Service Handbooks, No. 2, London: Headley Brothers.

Newman, G. (1911), *Annual Report for 1910 of the Chief Medical Officer of the Board of Education*, London: HMSO.
Newman, G. (1915), *Annual Report for 1914 of the Chief Medical Officer of the Board of Education*, London: HMSO.
Newman, G. (1920), *The Place of Public Opinion in Preventive Medicine*, London: HMSO.
Newman, G. (1925), *Public Education in Health*, London: HMSO.
Newman, G. (1939), *The Building of a Nation's Health*, London: Macmillan.
Orr, J. Boyd (1936), *Food, Health and Income: Report on a Survey of Diet in Relation to Income*, London: Macmillan.
Parliamentary Debates (Commons) (1935–6), *Malnutrition*, **314**, *c* 1229–1350.
Paton, D.N. and Findlay, L. (1926), *Child Life Investigations: Poverty, Nutrition and Growth*, Medical Research Council Special Report Series No. 101, London: HMSO.
Petty, C. (1987), 'The impact of the newer knowledge of nutrition: nutrition science and nutrition policy 1900–1939', Ph.D. thesis, London School of Hygiene and Tropical Medicine.
Petty, C. (1989), 'Primary research and public health: the prioritization of nutrition research in inter-war Britain', in Austoker, J. and Bryder, L. (eds), *Historical Perspectives on the role of the Medical Research Council*, London and Oxford: Oxford University Press.
Royal Commission on Physical Training (Scotland) (1903), *Report*, Vol. 1 Reports and Appendix, Cd 1507; Vol. 2 Evidence and Index, Cd 1508, London: HMSO.
Smith, D.F. (1986), 'Nutrition in Britain in the twentieth century', Ph.D. thesis, University of Edinburgh.
Smith, D. and Nicolson, M. (1989), 'The "Glasgow School" of Paton, Findlay and Cathcart: Conservative thought in chemical physiology, nutrition and public health', *Social Studies in Science*, **19**:195–238.
Thompson, E.P. (1967), 'Time, work-discipline and industrial capitalism', *Past and Present*, **37**:56–97.
Tomes, N. (1990), 'The private side of public health: sanitary science, domestic hygiene, and the germ theory, 1870–1900', *Bulletin of the History of Medicine*, **64**:509–39.
Townsend, P., Phillimore, P. and Beattie, A. (1986), *Inequalities in Health in the Northern Region: Interim Report*, Northern Regional Health Authority and the University of Bristol.
Townsend, P., Phillimore, P. and Beattie, A. (1988), *Health and Deprivation: Inequality and the North*, London: Croom Helm.
Turner, B.S. (1982a), 'The government of the body: medical regimens and the rationalization of diet', *British Journal of Sociology*, **33**:254–269.
Turner, B.S. (1982b), 'The discourse of diet', *Theory Culture and Society*, **1**:23–32.
Turner, B.S. (1985), 'More on "The government of the body": a reply to Naomi Aronson', *British Journal of Sociology*, **36**:151–3.
Turner, B.S. (1987), *Medical Power and Social Knowledge*, London: Sage.
Webster, C. (1982), 'Healthy or hungry Thirties?', *History Workshop*, **13**:110–29.
Webster, C. (1985), 'Health, welfare and unemployment during the Depression', *Past and Present*, **109**:204–230.

Williams, A.S. (1987), *The Rich Man and the Diseased Poor in Early Victorian Britain*, Basingstoke and London: Macmillan.
Wohl, A.S. (1983), *Endangered Lives: Public Health in Victorian Britain*, Cambridge, Massachusetts: Harvard University Press.

Index

For Product Safety Concerns and Information please contact our EU representative GPSR@taylorandfrancis.com
Taylor & Francis Verlag GmbH, Kaufingerstraße 24, 80331 München, Germany

www.ingramcontent.com/pod-product-compliance
Ingram Content Group UK Ltd.
Pitfield, Milton Keynes, MK11 3LW, UK
UKHW021512250926
475702UK00043B/41
* 9 7 8 0 8 1 5 3 4 8 6 2 7 *